THE GLOBAL MENTAL HEALTHCARE CRISIS

THE GLOBAL MENTAL HEALTHCARE CRISIS

TRANSITIONING FROM INSTITUTIONALIZATION TO COMMUNITY-BASED TREATMENT

FIRST EDITION

DELIA MARIE FRANKLIN, RN

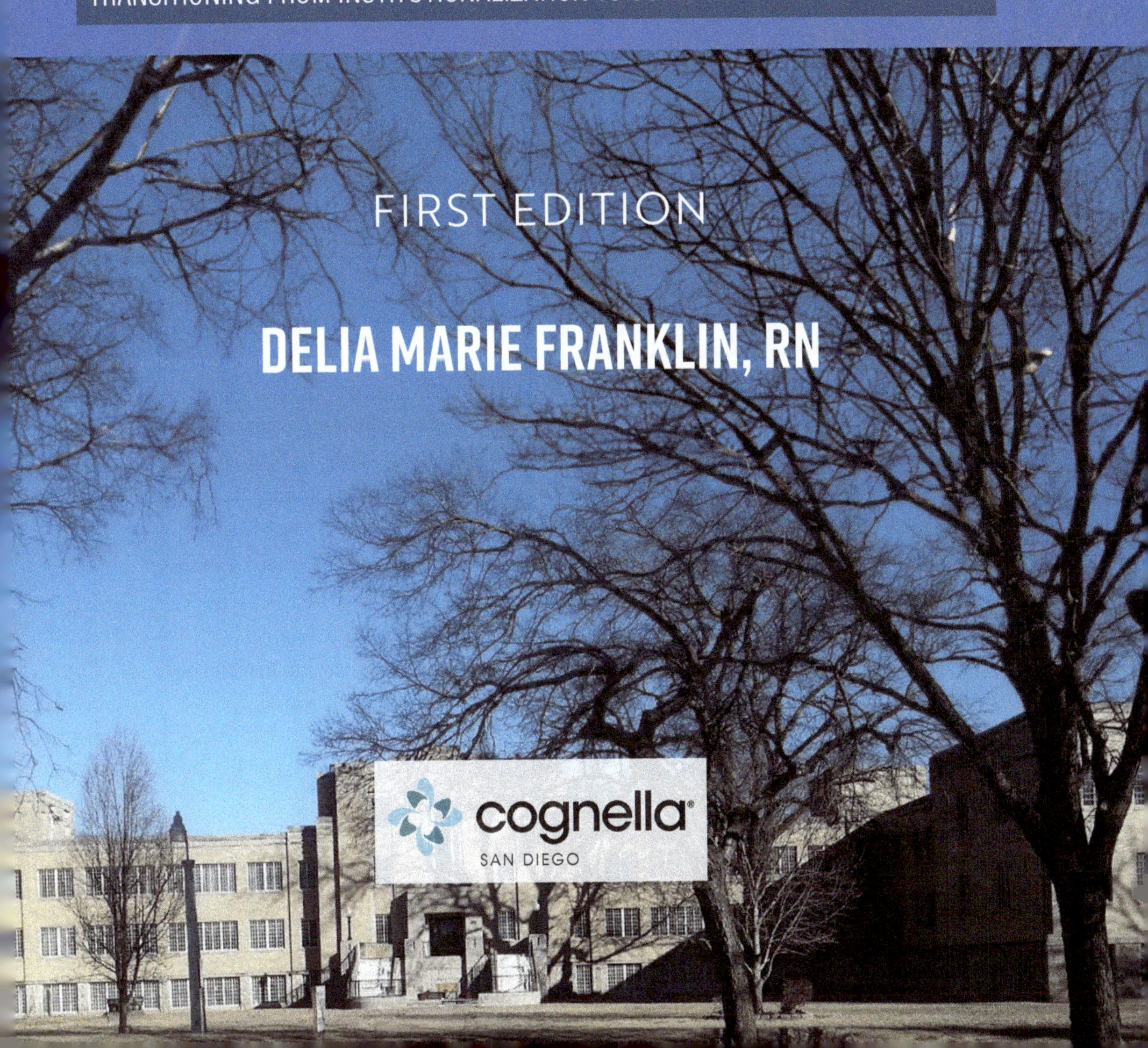

cognella®
SAN DIEGO

Bassim Hamadeh, CEO and Publisher
Amanda Martin, Executive Publisher
Amy Smith, Senior Project Editor
Jeanine Rees, Production Editor
Emely Villavicencio, Senior Graphic Designer
Kylie Bartolome, Licensing Specialist
Natalie Piccotti, Director of Marketing
Kassie Graves, Senior Vice President, Editorial

Printed in the United States of America.

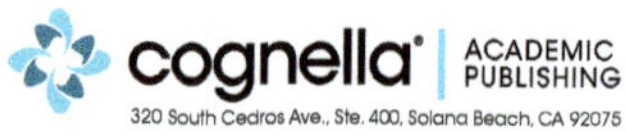

The Global Mental Healthcare Crisis: Transitioning From Institutionalization to Community-Based Treatment is dedicated to all of the health care providers who have been injured or killed while serving the mentally ill and all the patients who have been mistreated and/or harmed over the centuries while institutionalized.

BRIEF CONTENTS

DETAILED CONTENTS

REVIEWERS

Cene' L. Livingston, DNP, APRN, PMHNP-BC, FNP-BC, CNE
Chair of Advanced Practice Programs
Oklahoma City University – Kramer School of Nursing

Marcia H. Ford, MSW, LCSW, Professor of Practice
George Warren Brown School of Social Work, Washington University in St. Louis

Dr. Andrea J. Kirk-Jenkins
Western Kentucky University

INTRODUCTION

The evolution of mental health care and its treatment modalities is controversial; both medical and psychological interventions actually began in the 18th century and have expanded and improved over the years through data obtained from psychiatric research cases. The incorporation of evidence-based, scientifically obtained practices into the psychiatric community is assisting in changing perceptions of mental illness within society. Unfortunately, stigma and discrimination toward individuals experiencing mental illnesses continues today, but it is not as drastic as first displayed in the 18th and 19th centuries.

While progressing through our discussion of mental healthcare delivery systems, the reader should try to be open-minded about the advancement of treatment modalities. Some of the earlier interventions and treatments are barbaric, but it is only through mistakes and successes that this spectrum of health care has progressed throughout the world. Historical psychiatric education is presented in some of the chapters to assist the reader to better understand where we are today in the provision of mental health services. Looking at where we have been in the past in this branch of medicine can assist in obtaining a foundation of improvement in mental well-being for individuals globally through developing systems that focus on the prevention, recovery, and stabilization of mental conditions.

As a nurse, the author spent 10 years of her career employed as a licensed practical nurse in a psychiatric institution. The hospital consisted of a psychiatric building, a substance use disorder facility, a detox and psychiatric medical-surgical unit, and two units for developmentally disabled children. During the time the author worked as a psychiatric nurse (1980s–1990s), there were many changes implemented regarding treatment modalities used in mental health care.

There were high doses of Thorazine® and Haldol® ordered and administered in psychiatric institutions in the 1980s; over time, the doses decreased, and clients' side effects were less apparent. Also, as alternate psychotropic medications were developed, the older medications were replaced with newer medications that exhibited fewer side effects.

The utilization of restraints (five-point leather, seclusion rooms, and camisoles) was a common occurrence also in the 1980s and 1990s, but over the years, the frequency and duration of utilization declined. An increase in safety protocols and monitoring in relation to restraints and psychotropic medications was also implemented over time, decreasing the potential for adverse outcomes.

By the late 20th century, more and more therapeutic interventions consisting of psychotherapy, group therapy, recreational therapy, and art therapy expanded.

The psychiatric hospital became a more humane environment for the treatment of individuals experiencing mental illness.

Through education, more individuals in society are beginning to comprehend that mental conditions are really no different than physical illness. Individuals diagnosed with serious mental illnesses that have a genetic predisposition cannot change or prevent their disease from occurring, just as an individual diagnosed with diabetes, hypothyroidism, or renal disease cannot. Mental health conditions require interventions of medications and therapies, which is no different than a physical condition or disorder within the human body. As we continue to evolve in our social perceptions related to the understanding of psychological illnesses, hopefully, acceptance of individuals diagnosed with these diseases will continue to increase, assisting them in contributing to our intellectual growth in the world.

Over the years, it has become increasingly apparent that the United States and other countries are in the middle of a mental healthcare crisis. There are multiple causes that have contributed to the decrease in the availability of treatment services for those experiencing mental illness, with one being the global closing of state-funded psychiatric hospitals. There is a growing body of data that is being evaluated with regard to the closing of psychiatric hospitals globally, and it is being debated whether the transition to community versus inpatient treatment for mental health conditions has been beneficial for the client or society.

In this book, discussion is presented on global mental healthcare systems by examining institutionalization, deinstitutionalization, transinstitutionalization, community-based treatment, substance misuse provisions, mental health care providers, pandemics, and governmental strategies related to mental health, examining their effects on the client, the mental health continuum, and society. It has been voiced by many healthcare professionals that, to sustain mental well-being globally, we need to improve community-based mental healthcare systems worldwide to meet the needs of clients, families, communities, and society as a whole.

PART I

GLOBAL MENTAL HEALTH CARE STRATEGIES

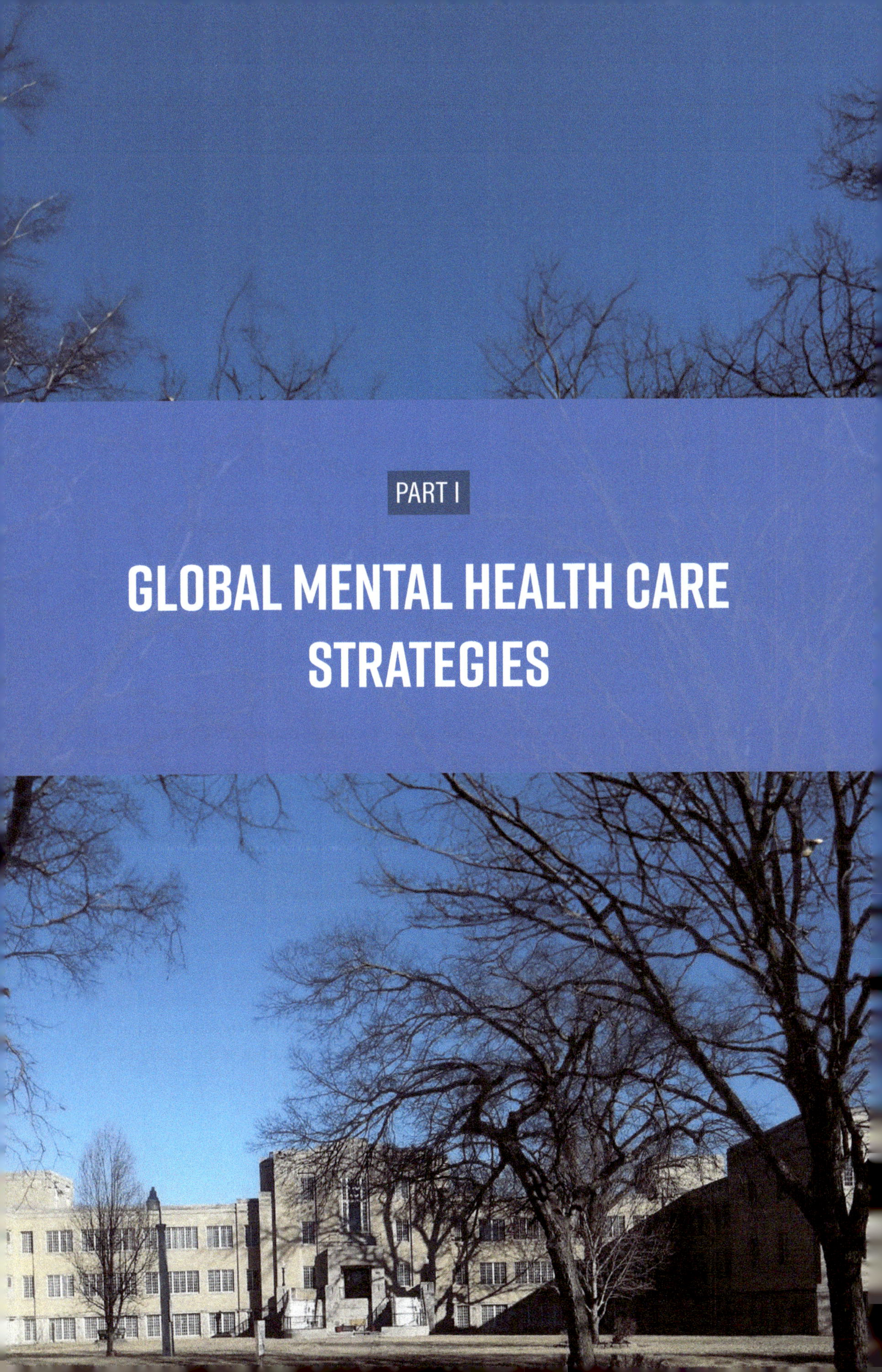

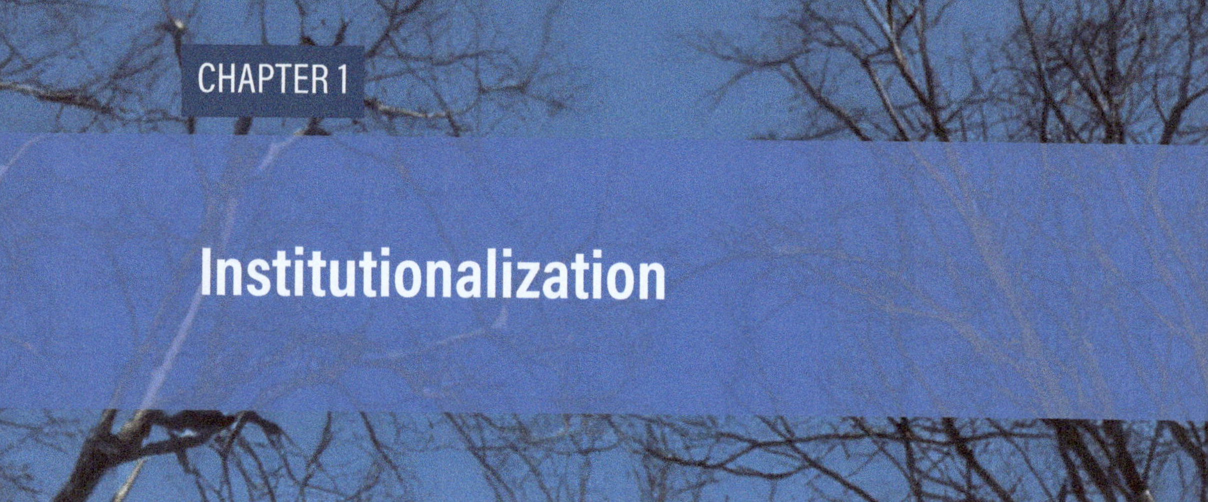

CHAPTER 1

Institutionalization

The main objective of this chapter is for the reader to gain a broader knowledge base about the worldwide institutionalization process to enhance understanding related to future mental health treatment systems implemented in countries.

In the 1800s, legal insanity was defined as "anything otherwise than normal." And psychiatric illnesses were classified as the following:

- Maniacal
- Melancholic
- Suicidal
- Homicidal tendencies

Attempts to collect data and measure the percentage of individuals with mental illness and mental retardation began in 1840 by the U.S. Census Bureau. The organization included the categories of "insane" and "idiotic" in their statistical data collection base.

During earlier centuries, psychiatric-diagnosed individuals were treated inhumanely by society and characterized as being "demon-possessed" or "crazed animals." In this time period, there was widespread utilization of physical, emotional, and psychological abuse against individuals classified as mentally ill. Plus, physical restraints, such as straitjackets and heavy chains, were used to control psychiatric patients during inpatient stays. Discussions in this chapter entail an examination of psychiatric institutions throughout the globe to enhance understanding of their construction and functionality, the laws implemented in countries that supported institutionalization, and modalities used for crisis intervention and mental health treatment during earlier centuries; a few are still in use today.

Laws

Involuntary admissions (civil commitments) to psychiatric hospitals in the United States were common practice in the 19th century. The National Mental Health Act of

1946 formulated the first mental health program in the United States to protect the rights of people experiencing mental illness. This program then led to the development of the National Institute of Mental Health (NIMH) in 1949 through generated funding that supported psychiatric research and education. In 1951, NIMH released a "Draft Act Governing Hospitalization of the Mentally Ill," calling for commitment decision-making to be returned to the medical profession.[1] Document 1.1 is a section of the annual report from a psychiatric hospital submitted to the governor of Nebraska in the early 1900s.

DOCUMENT 1.1 1906 Report "State Hospital for Insane." Nebraska Library Commission. The Atrium, 1200 N Street, Suite 120, Lincoln, Nebraska 68508-2023

Ninth Biennial Report of the State Hospital for Insane at Ingleside, Nebraska to the Governor for the Biennial Period Ending November 30, 1906

State Board of Control

Hon. H.M. Eaton	Commissioner Public Lands & Buildings
Hon. A Galusha	Secretary of State
Hon. Peter Mortensen	Treasurer of State
Hon. Norris Brown	Attorney General

Resident Officers

W.B. Kern, M.D.	Superintendent
H.C. Haverly	Steward

Medical Staff

W.B. Kern, M.D.	Superintendent
W.H. Chapman, M.D.	First Assistant Physician
A. Morefield, M.D.	Second Assistant Physician
F.P. Simms, M.D.	Third Assistant Physician
G.E. Spear, M.D.	Fourth Assistant Physician

To His Excellency, John H. Mickey, Governor of Nebraska:

Dear Sir.—In harmony with the legal and customary requirements I have the honor to submit herewith this, the Ninth Biennial Report of this Institution, The State Hospital for Insane, for the biennial period ending November 30th, 1906.

At the beginning of this biennial period, Dec. 1st, 1904, there were nine hundred eighty-seven (987) patients in the Institution, of whom six hundred sixty-seven (667) were males and three hundred twenty (320) were females. During the biennium, one hundred ninety-eight (198) have been admitted, of whom one hundred sixty-three (163) were males and thirty-five (35) were females. Of these six (6) were discharged as recovered, seventeen (17) improved, two (2) unimproved, thirty-three (33) paroled and one hundred seventy-one (171) died. During this period, two (2) patients have been transferred to the Lincoln Asylum.

During the period covered by this report the general health of the inmates has been exceptionally good. The modern sanitary and other appliances tending toward the health and comfort of the patients have been improved in many ways, and the Institution is nearer accomplishing that for which it was established, than ever before.

The per capita cost for the biennial period was two hundred eighty-seven dollars and fifty cents ($287.50), or an average daily per capita of thirty-nine and three-eighths cents (39 3/8c).

OCCUPATION

The great value of suitable occupation and employment for those who have passed the first stage of mental disease is well recognized, and a strong effort has been made in this hospital to provide such employment for those willing to be employed. A large number of patients have been regularly employed on the farm and in the gardens, dairy, laundry, sewing room, and other industrial departments. For the past few years we have been able to manufacture practically all the mattresses used in the Hospital. The sewing room has not only supplied all the clothing for the female department of the Institution, but for the past two years practically all the underwear required in the male department as well.

IMPROVEMENTS

During the biennial period just closed many substantial improvements have been made, the most important of these are as follows:

A new amusement hall building, on the first floor of which is located a general store room, drug room and sewing room. This is a handsome building and furnishes the Institution with an elegant auditorium sixty by one hundred feet, an improvement very much needed. A new farm cottage has been located one-half mile southwest of the Hospital which accommodates twenty-five (25) male patients, most of these being employed in the dairy department.

From a special appropriation made by the last legislature, two new greenhouses (each 24x120 ft.) have been built, and two new marine boilers, each two hundred fifty (250) horse power, have been installed; also one additional dynamo, 100 K. W. added to our lighting plant; and two additional Kirker-Bender fire escapes installed.

The entire exterior of the main building has recently been re-painted, and has not only materially benefited the buildings, but has greatly improved the general appearance of the Institution. The sewer has been extended about twenty-one hundred (2100) feet, and at this time empties at a point more than three quarters of a mile from the Institution. The lawn has been vastly increased in size during the biennium, and a large number of additional shade, fruit, and ornamental trees added. Forty thousand (40,000) square feet of manufactured stone walks have been laid and is one of the very noticeable and substantial improvements. Our gardens this year represented approximately one hundred thirty (130) acres and the yield was very abundant.

ENTERTAINMENTS

More than the usual amount of amusement and entertainment has been provided during the biennium, and especially so since the opening of our new amusement hall; usually one or two dances and one musical recital each week, in addition to frequent chapel services.

NEEDS OF THE INSTITUTION

The Institution is very much in need of another building for the care of female patients, and in addition to this, a good modern isolation cottage with a capacity of from seventy to one hundred beds, for the care of tubercular and other contagious and infectious diseases. Additional coal bins, or room for storing coal, is greatly needed and for the purpose of erecting such a building, an appropriation of five thousand dollars ($5,000) is asked.

The offices in the Administration Building being quite inadequate for an Institution of this size, it is certainly advisable to provide additional room in this department, hence it is recommended that a suitable cottage be erected to be used as a residence by the superintendent and bis family and the rooms at present used for this purpose be converted into offices. The number of night watches, night nurses and other night employees has of necessity increased in number until it is very necessary to provide desirable apartments for them and a detached building of suitable size to be used as a night watch cottage is also recommended and very much needed.

CONCLUSION

In conclusion I wish to express my earnest appreciation of the loyalty and fidelity of our esteemed steward, Mr. H. C. Haverly, whose valuable assistance is most highly appreciated. Also to extend my sincere thanks to those constituting the assistant physicians on our medical staff, who have so faithfully and intelligently performed their respective duties; and to the various heads of the departments and other employees who have lent much valuable assistance in the success of the Institution.

To Your Excellency, the Governor, and the Board of Public Lands and Buildings, I desire to assure you of my appreciation of your kindly and loyal assistance and your constant and valuable advice.

Respectfully,

W. B. KERN, M. D., Superintendent.

Nebraska Library Commission, Ninth Biennial Report of the State Hospital for Insane at Ingleside, Nebraska to the Governor, 1906.

NIMH presented a strategic plan of goals in 2020, including defining the brain mechanisms underlying complex behaviors, examining mental illness trajectories across the life span, striving for prevention and cures, and strengthening the public health impact of NIMH-supported research.[2]

United Kingdom

Other countries, like the United Kingdom, passed laws through parliament, such as the Madhouses Act of 1774 and the Lunacy Act of 1845. The Madhouses Act set a legal framework for regulating insane asylums, referred to as "madhouses" in the United Kingdom during the 18th century. The institutions had to be licensed, inspected annually, and maintain a roster of all patients residing in the "madhouse." The Lunacy Act was implemented in conjunction with the County Asylums Act of 1845 and essentially changed the categorization of those experiencing mental conditions to the status of a patient.

Italy

In 1865, Italy put in place the City and Province Law no. 2248 that instituted governments to take care of individuals experiencing mental illness. Also, an Italian 1904 Law no. 36 explained that individuals with a mental illness must be treated in mental hospitals when dangerous to themselves or others or when creating a public scandal. Law 180, or Basaglia Law, was implemented in 1978 and is the Italian Mental Health Act that initiated the closing of all state-funded psychiatric institutions in Italy.[3]

Canada

Ontario passed an act (SUC, 1839, Chap. XI) in 1839 to institute the construction of an asylum within the province for the insane and lunatic person. Prior to 1845, the care of individuals experiencing mental illness in many Canadian Provinces was mostly supported by religious authorities and police. It is believed that the first Hotel Dieu was founded in Quebec City in 1639 by the Duchess d'Aiguillon and was used to treat indigent patients, the crippled, and idiots. Dr. Clarence M. Hincks and Clifford Beers organized the Canadian National Committee for Mental Hygiene in 1918.[4] The health organization is currently called the Canadian Mental Health Association and is the oldest operating health institution in Canada. The Canadian Mental Health Act, which used five previous mental health laws, was established in 1965.

France

In 1838, France passed its first law on hospital admissions for individuals experiencing mental illness. The Law of June 30th, 1838, also known as the law on the insane (loi sur les alienes), allowed for all people to be hospitalized without their consent.

In June of 1990, the law was amended to incorporate voluntary admissions as the standard of practice versus involuntary admissions to psychiatric hospitals.[5] The law subsequently had additional revisions and clarifications in 2011 and 2013; the last law explains the role of the judge in psychiatric hospital admission processes.

Psychiatric Institutions

Psychiatric hospitals have existed for centuries globally and were referred to as "lunatic asylums" until around the 20th century, when modern belief systems and treatment modalities began to emerge, altering the medical community's perceptions of mental illness. During medieval time frames, other names were attached to lunatic asylums, such as monasteries, fool's towers, and Hotel Dieus. Mental health institutions have also been associated with other titles over the years, including the following:

- Lunatic hospitals
- Insane asylums
- Mental health centers
- Regional centers
- Asylums for the insane
- Retreats

By the year 1840, eight "lunatic asylums" existed in the United States. From 1840 to 1900, individuals such as Dorothea Dix, an American reformer, increased awareness of the necessity of specialized hospitals to house clients experiencing mental illness, resulting in the construction or expansion of 32 mental hospitals. The majority of state psychiatric hospitals were originally built under the "Kirkbride Plan," which was formulated by Dr. Thomas Story Kirkbride through his 1845 book *On the Construction, Organization, and General Arrangements of Hospitals for the Insane.*[6]

Dr. Kirkbride served his patients in a humane and compassionate manner and structured the architectural design of psychiatric hospitals in a linear fashion, which he believed restored patients to a more natural balance by providing fresh air and natural lighting. "Moral treatment" was the philosophy instituted and practiced by Dr. Kirkbride and his followers.[7] During this historical era, practitioners believed that isolating patients from their causes of insanity would be beneficial in curing them, thus hopefully decreasing mental illness within society. Most state psychiatric institutions were built between 1850 to 1860 and were geographically isolated to decrease political opposition to mental health institution construction.

Under the Kirkbride Plan, early psychiatric institutions were structured to provide work for patients, including farms, sewing rooms, janitorial duties, etc. It was believed during this era that keeping the mind engaged while providing a healthy environment would assist patients in recovering from their mental illness and returning to society. Because of a lack of documentation to substantiate that this process promoted or maintained recovery from psychosis or mental illness, the Kirkbride Plan was eliminated when other treatment modalities became available in the United States.

Mental Institutions in the United States

During the 18th century (1773) in Williamsburg, Virginia, the first hospital for psychiatric treatment was constructed and opened: Eastern State Hospital. The process of building Eastern State Hospital is largely attributed to Governor Francis Fauquier, who addressed legislature about the treatment of mentally ill clients. Psychiatric treatment of patients continues at Eastern State Hospital in a facility on the outskirts of Williamsburg, Virginia. The new facility is accredited by the Joint Commission and includes 16 buildings and houses 317 beds. Eastern State Hospital's mission and vision for their institution are the following:

> Our **MISSION** is to partner with those we serve to promote personal independence. Our **VISION** is to continuously pursue the highest quality services that empower individuals in their recovery.[8]

The first private psychiatric hospital in the United States opened in Philadelphia, Pennsylvania, in 1813; Friends Asylum for the Relief of Persons Deprived of the Use of Their Reason. The Quakers followed Dr. Kirkbride's treatment of care for those experiencing mental conditions of "moral treatment." It was the belief system of the Quaker religion that "insanity was merely another obstacle to be removed from the road to inward enlightenment, and like slavery and poverty, was curable."[9]

Pilgrim State Hospital

Pilgrim State Hospital is located in Brentwood, New York, on 1,900 acres of land and is believed to be the largest psychiatric institution to have ever been in existence. The original architectural design was constructed between 1930 and 1941, consisting of approximately 27 buildings that could house 12,000 patients.[10] Opening its doors for clients in 1941, the institution consisted of a medical hospital, laboratories, consultation rooms, a nursing school, pathology departments, a theater, a bakery, laundry services, a firehouse, a power plant, employee and nurse's housing, a cemetery, and a community farm.

A veteran's hospital named Mason General Hospital was built next to Pilgrim State Hospital in 1944, operating until 1946 in a veteran capacity. Three of the buildings from Mason General were given to Pilgrim State Hospital in the late 1940s, increasing the client population to 15,000 during that time frame.[11]

Pilgrim State Hospital is currently abandoned, but during its operating years, it provided insulin shock therapy, Metrazol® shock therapy, and electric shock therapy. Frontal lobotomies were initiated in 1946, and as many as 2,000 lobotomy procedures were performed at this hospital during the surgical procedure's existence. The lobotomy procedure was generally used with severely violent patients. In the 1950s, Thorazine became publicly available in the medical community for the treatment of psychiatric conditions, decreasing the utilization of some of the controversial procedures in these institutions.

Trans-Allegheny Lunatic Asylum

Located in Weston, West Virginia, the Trans-Allegheny Lunatic Asylum (Weston State Hospital) was constructed from 1858 to 1881, opening for patient admissions in 1864. The building is an original Kirkbride design that is still standing and currently serves as a tourist attraction, being one of the largest hand-cut stone masonry buildings in the United States. The hospital ceased operating as a mental health treatment facility for patients in 1994 because of the construction of a new psychiatric hospital.

The facility was originally designed to house 250 patients, but by the 1950s, there were an estimated 2,600 patients being treated at the hospital. Because of the overcrowding, the Trans-Allegheny Lunatic Asylum became the leader in the "West Virginia Lobotomy Project" led by Dr. Walter Freeman. The transorbital lobotomy was used throughout the United States in psychiatric hospitals that were overpopulated and understaffed and is discussed in more detail later in this chapter.

It is publicly believed that the institution experiences paranormal activity, and ghost hunt tours are available at the asylum. The asylum has been featured on *Ghost Stories, Syfy's Ghost Hunters,* and the *Travel Channel's Ghost Adventures.* The author personally experienced and toured this facility in 2022 and captured an apparition in one of the photos taken during the tour. You can decide for yourself; no alterations have been made to Figure 1.1, except the removal of the other tourists in the photograph. Some individuals who reside in this area believe that the controversial treatment modalities used over the centuries at the psychiatric institution have resulted in spirits being trapped, unable to transcend to alternate destinations. This leads to the question, Is there really an astral plane?

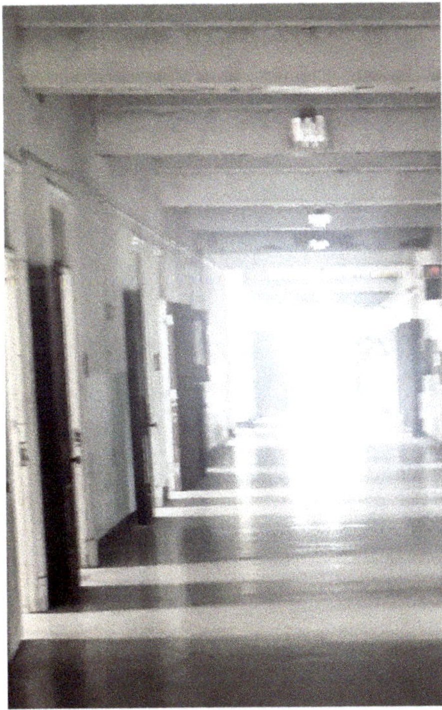

FIGURE 1.1 Apparition Trans-Allegheny Lunatic Asylum

The restoration of the Trans-Allegheny Lunatic Asylum is partially funded by the several different tours offered at the National Historic Landmark (1990). Figures 1.2 to 1.5 are pictures of the Trans-Allegheny Lunatic Asylum located in Weston, West

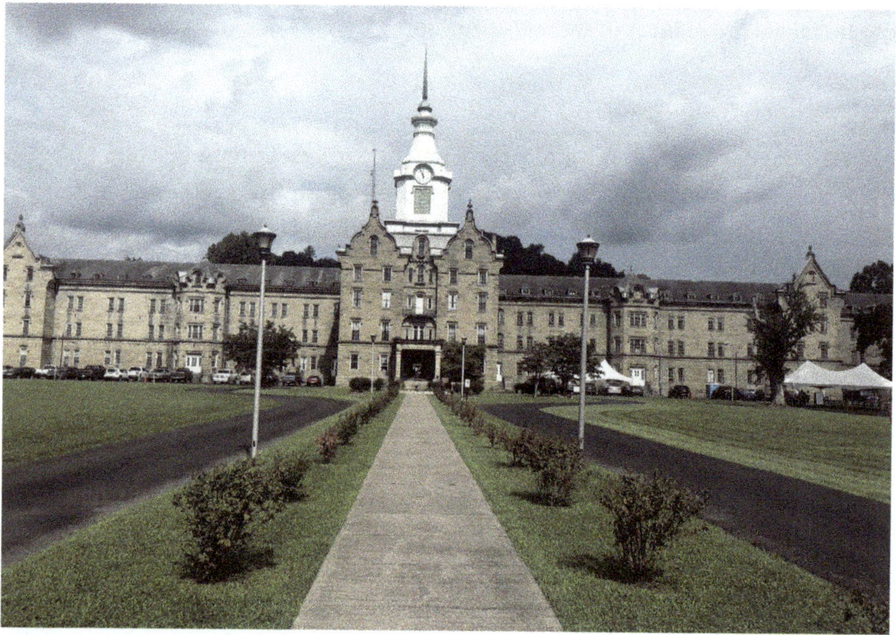

FIGURE 1.2 Trans-Allegheny Lunatic Asylum

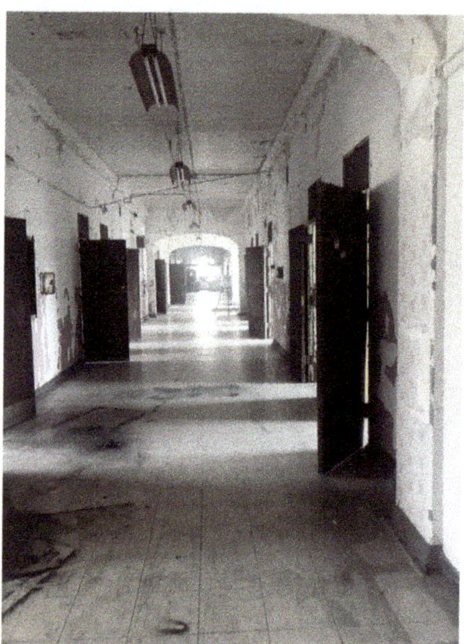

FIGURE 1.3 Hallway Trans-Allegheny Lunatic Asylum

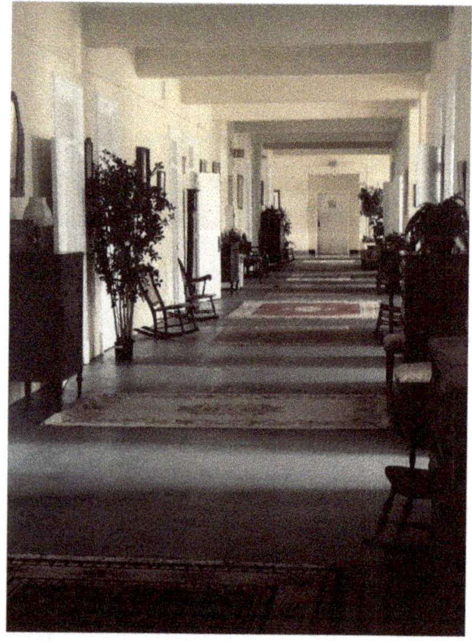

FIGURE 1.4 Restoration Trans-Allegheny Lunatic Asylum

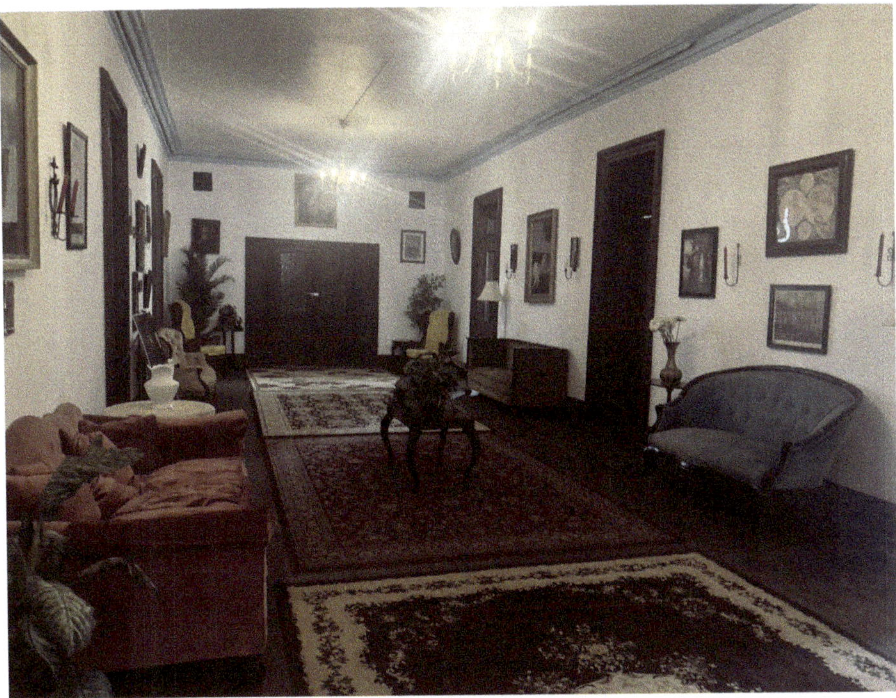

FIGURE 1.5 Restoration Trans-Allegheny Lunatic Asylum

Virginia. Employees dress for the time period of early operation of the mental hospital and provide information on architecture, history, paranormal activity, mental health treatment modalities, and institutional-specific practices. This institution provides insight into the history of mental health care in the United States.

McLean Hospital

This hospital was originally named the "Asylum for the Insane" when constructed in 1811 on acres of land in a section of Charlestown, Massachusetts. Complete construction of the hospital was finalized by 1818; several other names were attributed to the hospital between 1811 and 1818, including Somerville Asylum and Charlestown Asylum. The name McLean Hospital was developed and implemented in 1892 in recognition of an early benefactor, Mr. John McLean. The hospital campus was moved to Belmont, Massachusetts, in 1895 because of new developmental projects in Charlestown.

In 1882, McLean established the first psychiatric training school for nurses. McLean Hospital is the largest psychiatric facility of Harvard Medical School and is known for its expertise and groundbreaking neuroscience research.[12] McLean Hospital has served in treating several famous individuals, including John Nash, James Taylor, Ray Charles, Susanna Kaysen, and David Foster Wallace. As a leader in psychiatric institutions, McLean Hospital provides teaching, treatment, and research, which sustains the hospital's existence and reputation.

Hastings Regional Center

This "State Asylum for the Incurably Insane" was constructed in 1887 on 160 acres of land by the town of Hastings, Nebraska. Charles C. Rittenhouse, a Hastings architect, developed the plans for the building, which was a three-story brick structure with a central tower. It was constructed due to overcrowding in the psychiatric institution located in Lincoln, Nebraska. When it opened its doors for patient admissions, the hospital received 44 patients from the Lincoln Asylum in 1889.[13] The original building had two new wings added in 1891, and it is no longer in existence.[14] In December of 1916, the facility housed 1,152 patients. Figures 1.6 and 1.7 are the originally constructed buildings at Hastings Regional Center (HRC) that have been demolished.

Over the years, the hospital expanded through the construction of a medical-surgical building, a psychiatric hospital, greenhouses, a chapel, an amusement hall, employee living quarters and an administration building. There are approximately 1,000 bodies buried in the institution's cemetery marked with numbers only to identify the individuals, with the last burial occurring in 1956. The institution participated in many mental health treatment modalities over the years, with electroshock therapy initiated in the 1920s. In the 1930s, fever therapy, hydrotherapy, and insulin shock therapy were used to treat patients. When psychoactive medications emerged in the 1950s, treatment modalities were altered, and patients received occupational therapy, psychotherapy, behavioral modification programs, recreational therapy, transactional analysis, and religious therapy programs.

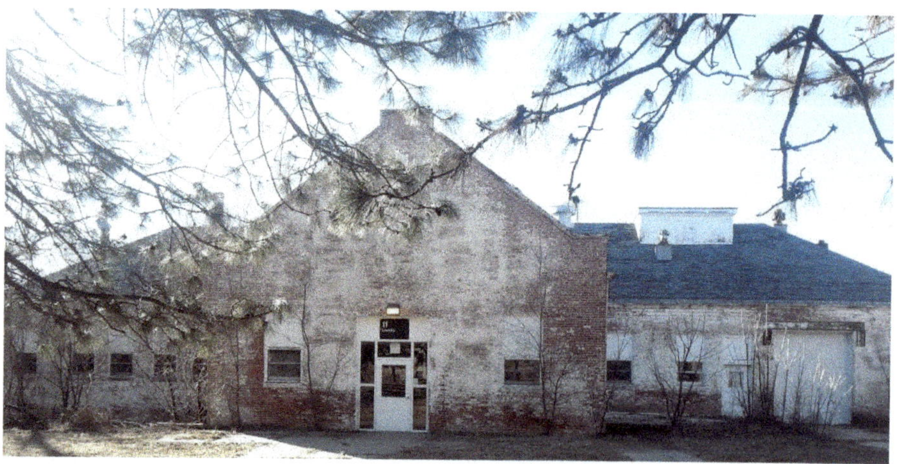

FIGURE 1.6 Original Laundry Building. (Early 1900s) HRC. 4200 West 2nd Street, Hastings, Nebraska 68901

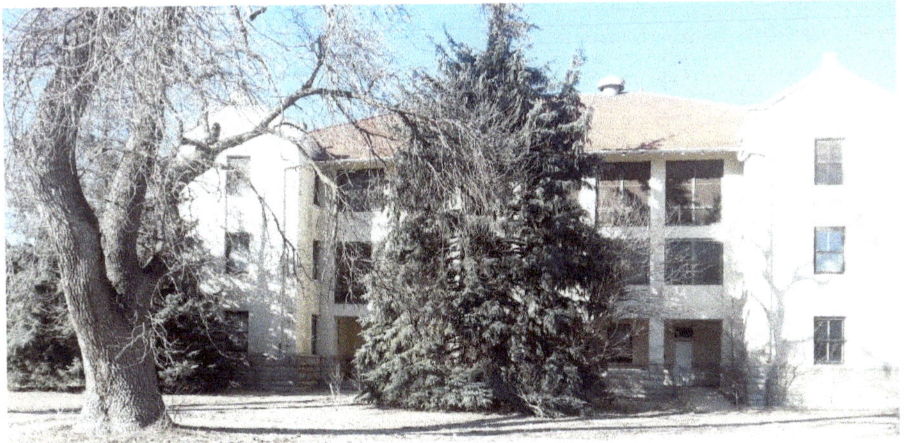

FIGURE 1.7 Original Tuberculosis Building (1910) HRC. 4200 West 2nd, Street Hastings, Nebraska 68901

In 1971, the institution changed its name for the sixth time to the "HRC." The institution was reorganized into two separate entities in 1963: a psychiatric and substance use disorder treatment hospital. In 2018, the institution was used as a Juvenile Chemical Dependency Treatment Center, with only one to three of its buildings open.

Approval was obtained for a demolition process of six of the institution's buildings in April of 2020. In April of 2022, the agenda was established to demolish the remainder of the buildings on the grounds, with an anticipated completion date in the summer of 2022. Figures 1.8, 1.9, and 1.10 are buildings that have been or are scheduled to be demolished.

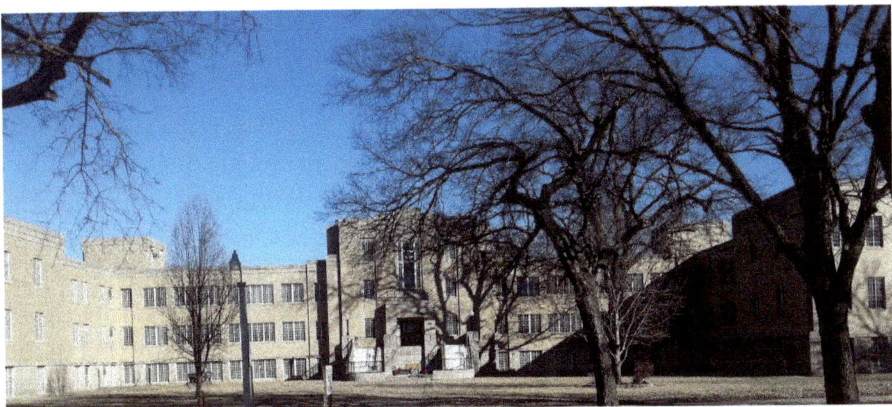

FIGURE 1.8 Building #3 Psychiatric Unit. (1938) HRC. 4200 West 2nd Street, Hastings, Nebraska 68901

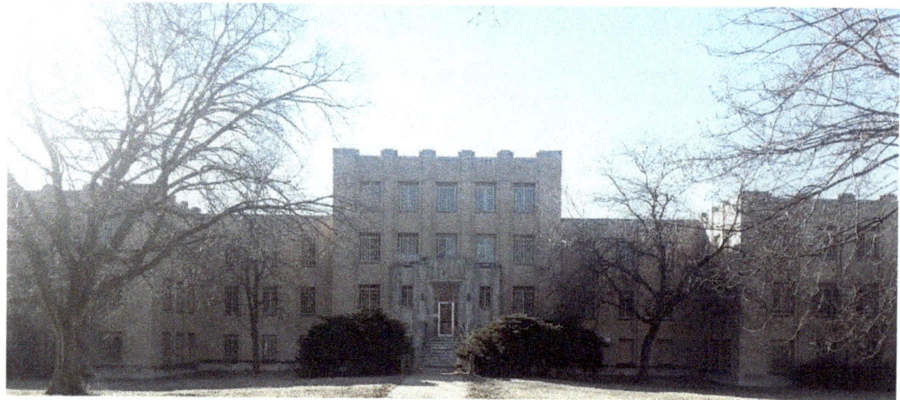

FIGURE 1.9 Building #7 Substance Abuse Program Unit. (1940s) HRC. 4200 West 2nd Street, Hastings, Nebraska 68901

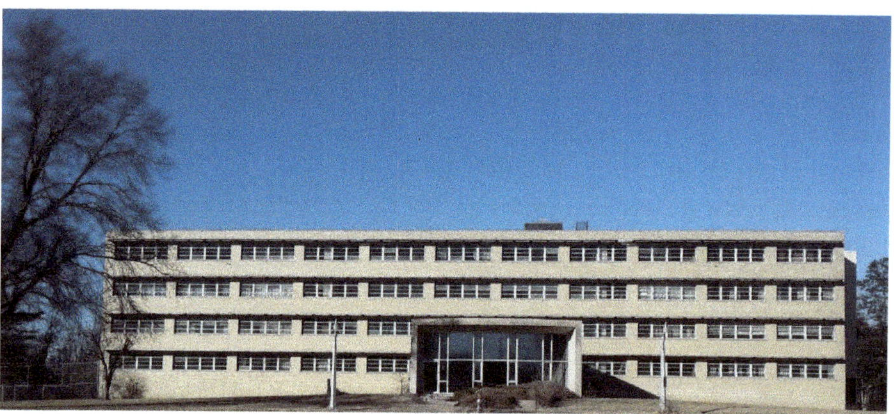

FIGURE 1.10 Building #4 Medical-Surgical Unit (1950s) HRC. 4200 West 2nd Street, Hastings, Nebraska 68901

NAPA State Hospital

Considered California's oldest state hospital still in operation, Napa State Hospital opened its doors on November 15, 1875, on a 138-acre campus. The original Kirkbride building, resembling a castle, was torn down after World War II. Currently, the hospital contains approximately 1,225 beds and does not accept voluntary admissions. Patients are admitted by civil commitment under the Lanterman-Petris-Short Act: Incompetent to Stand Trial (PC 1370), Offenders with Mental Health Disorders (Penal code section/2972), and Not Guilty by Reason of Insanity (PC 1026). The facility is accredited by the Joint Commission on Accreditation of Healthcare Organizations. Notable patients that have resided at the institution include Edward Charles Allaway (mass murderer), Eddie Machen (boxer, threatened suicide), Earle Nelson (serial killer), and Scott Harlan Thorpe (spree killer).[15]

Mental Institutions in Other Countries

Located in Italy, the Mombello Psychiatric Hospital was the largest asylum in Italy, officially established in 1878. Mombello was a previously constructed building that was renovated from 1873 to 1878, but it initiated admitting patients in 1865. By 1867, Mombello housed around 300 patients. The patients were categorized by attitude and behavior: the quiet ones, the agitated ones, the filthy ones, and the workers. The facility was perceived as being its own village and even produced its own newspaper between the years of 1880 to 1905. During World War I, the facility housed approximately 3,000 patients. Many famous doctors were employed by the facility; two of those were Ugo Cerletti, the inventor of electroconvulsive therapy, and Gaetano Perusini, colleague and pupil of psychiatrist Alois Alzheimer. Mombello is currently an abandoned building that was officially closed in 1978.[16]

Bethlem

England's first psychiatric hospital, Bethlem, was originally constructed as a general hospital in 1247. By 1403, the majority of the patients at Bethlem were those experiencing mental illness. It is reported that corporal punishment, some barbaric treatments, and isolation were used at the facility. The facility was rebuilt in 1676 and described as looking more like Versailles versus a mental hospital.

This psychiatric hospital was used as a tourist attraction in the 17th and 18th centuries; the practice was terminated in 1770. In 1815, the Versailles version of the psychiatric hospital was torn down, and a new facility was constructed.[17] Today, the facility is a psychiatric hospital called Bethlem Royal Hospital that provides services for learning disabilities, geriatric psychiatry, forensic psychiatry, child and adolescent psychiatry, and adult mental illness.

Orilla Asylum

Located in Canada, the psychiatric institution opened its doors in 1876 as the "Asylum for Idiots." In 1907, the psychiatric hospital was renamed the Ontario Hospital. Most admissions to Orilla came from welfare institutions, including the Children's Aid Society, Toronto General Hospital, Mental Hygiene Clinic, and various orphanages. Orilla Asylum was populated with both children and adults for whom the institution became a life-long place of residence. Overcrowding generated public concern about the institution in the 1960s, and a movement toward deinstitutionalization was implemented. The institution was again renamed in 1973 as the Huronia Regional Centre. Ontario developed a 5-year closure plan for Orilla in 1975 and completed the task in 2009.[18]

Charenton

Founded as a lunatic asylum in 1645 by Freres de la Charite, Charenton was a catholic institution located in France. It was known for the humane treatment of its patients, with an emphasis on art therapy. In September of 1660, individuals experiencing mental illnesses were required to be cared for in hospitals per French government mandate. This hospital housed some famous individuals: Jerome-Joseph de Momigny, a Belgian musicologist and composer who died in the institution in 1842; Andre Gill, a caricaturist who died in the institution in 1885; and Andre Bloch, a mathematician who spent the last 3 decades of his life at Charenton. In 1991, the institution became a public hospital.[19] Some of the clients admitted to psychiatric institutions during earlier centuries addressed reform measures on behalf of patients' rights; one of those people was Clifford Beers.

Clifford Beers

Clifford Beers was a Wall Street Financier who graduated from Yale College and suffered a mental breakdown with a subsequent suicide attempt in the early 1900s. Mr. Beers spent several years institutionalized because of his diagnosis of bipolar disorder and was subjected to inhumane treatment in the hospitals he was seeking help from during his life. During his stay in mental institutions, Mr. Beers, at one point, was confined to a straitjacket for 21 consecutive nights.[20] After being released from a psychiatric hospital in 1908, Mr. Beers wrote and published his book, *A Mind That Found Itself.*

The book led to mental health care reform in the United States and other countries, instituting the National Committee for Mental Hygiene in 1909, currently called the National Mental Health Association. The goals of the organization in the early 1900s were as follows:

- To improve attitudes toward mental illness and the mentally ill
- To improve services for the mentally ill
- To work toward the prevention of mental illness and promote mental health[21]

The following report in Document 1.2 depicts the gender specifics of psychiatric institutional admissions.

In 1930, Mr. Beers formulated the first International Congress for Mental Hygiene, leading to the establishment of the International Committee for Mental Hygiene, currently known as the World Federation for Mental Health. The first outpatient mental health clinic was developed by Mr. Beers (Clifford Beers Clinic), located in New Haven, Connecticut, in 1913. During his lifetime, Mr. Beers worked on improving the quality of treatment and care for those experiencing mental conditions throughout the United States and the world. Mr. Beers died in 1943.

DOCUMENT 1.2 1906 Report "State Hospital for Insane" Nebraska Library Commission, the Atrium.

MONTHLY ADMISSION OF PATIENTS

Admitted during the Biennial Period ending November 30th, 1906.

Months—	Males	Females	Total
December, 1904	0	2	2
January, 1905	24	0	24
April, 1905	2	0	2
May, 1905	0	2	2
June, 1905	1	1	2
July, 1905	1	0	1
August, 1905	25	0	25
October, 1905	4	1	5
November, 1905	0	1	1
December, 1905	42	15	57
February, 1906	0	1	1
April, 1906	1	0	1
May, 1906	31	12	43
June, 1906	2	0	2
September, 1906	2	0	2
October, 1906	28	0	28
Totals	**163**	**35**	**198**

Nebraska Library Commission, Ninth Biennial Report of the State Hospital for Insane at Ingleside, Nebraska to the Governor, 1906.

Mr. Beers led the path to improve the quality of care in psychiatric hospitals, yet even with all his efforts, problems still existed. In April of 1969, the Pennsylvania state public welfare secretary, John F. White, formed a special task force to investigate Byberry State Hospital, a now-closed state institution with one of the most horrifying records of patient death and abuse. In September of that year, the group issued a report in which it said that patients were being neglected, beaten, and sexually abused. The report called for "immediate and drastic action to reverse the history of neglect, poor management, absence of treatment and rampant abuse."[22] Mistreatment of patients, as addressed by Mr. Beers in 1908, included crisis intervention modalities in behavioral health hospitals and institutions that are still being evaluated today.

Crisis Intervention Modalities

Although seclusion and restraints have been used for centuries in psychiatric institutions, they have been scrutinized for some time due to the number of reported cases that result in injury and death annually while using these procedural interventions. Advocates against seclusion and restraints argue that the procedures need to be psychologically viewed as a form of abuse toward patients, such as assault and battery, and that the procedures are a human rights violation.

A 2018 study revealed that over 80% of psychiatric and general hospitals still report the utilization of seclusion and restraint practices.[23] It is further argued that the continued acceptance of violence within society contributes to the institutionalization of accepted violence in the mental health profession, which includes some of the past and present treatment modalities used with psychiatric patients around the world.

The World Health Organization launched a training program, "Strategies to End Seclusion and Restraints," in 2019. The organization acknowledges that seclusion and restraints are widely prevalent practices in mental health care worldwide, which generate physical and mental harm to patients. A 2016 study of four similar European countries revealed the percentage of patients exposed to restraints varied from 4.5% to 9.4%, the average number of restraints per patient was around three episodes in all countries, the Netherlands had the highest use of seclusion at 79% and the longest restraint times, Wales had the lowest use of seclusion at 2%, and Germany exhibited a 49% rate of seclusion utilization.[24]

Seclusion

According to the Centers for Medicare and Medicaid Services (CMS), seclusion is defined as the involuntary confinement of a patient alone in a room or area from which the patient is physically prevented from leaving. Seclusion may be implemented only for the management of violent or self-destructive behavior.[25] The practice has been used in psychiatric settings and society since ancient Greek and Roman time frames. Current recommendations for psychiatric hospital seclusion rooms are as follows:

- Allows for communication with the patient (intercom)
- Has limited furnishings
- No safety hazards
- Robust, reinforced windows that allow natural light
- Robust doors that open outward
- No blind spots (viewing panels or CCTV)
- Has a clock that is always visible to the patient
- Has externally controlled heating and air conditioning[26]

The Department of Health and Human Services, Health Care Financing Administration released a paper in 1999 stating that all clients placed in seclusion or restraint must be assessed by a physician or state-approved licensed practitioner within 1 hour of initiation of the procedure to ensure the procedure is warranted and properly implemented. No form of seclusion or restraint will be used as a form of coercion, discipline, convenience, or retaliation. And any death that results while a client is secluded or restrained will be reported to the Health and Human Services Department, which will in turn be reported to the state Protection and Advocacy Agencies. Figure 1.11 demonstrates seclusion episodes in psychiatric hospitals.

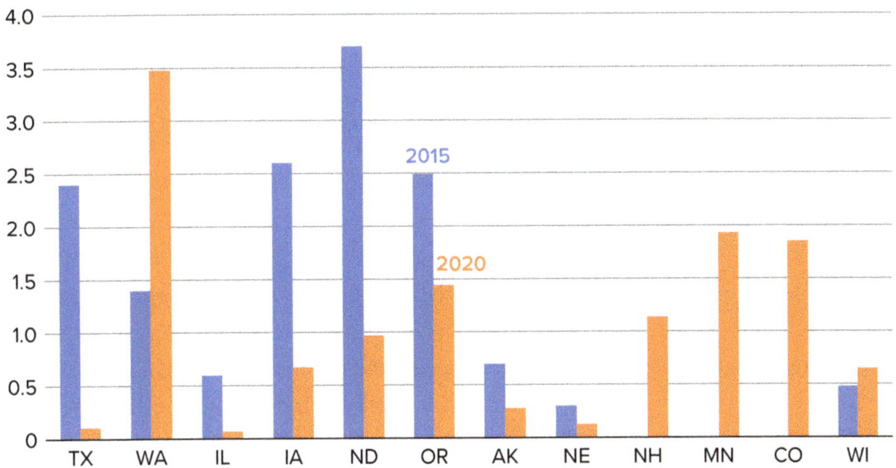

FIGURE 1.11 Seclusion Episodes 2015 And 2020 (Overall Rate per 1000)[27]

Data collected by CMS in 2015 and 2020 revealed a decrease in seclusion utilization hours by 120,588 (2015—309,951 hours; 2020—189,363 hours) in U.S. psychiatric settings.[28]

The Bureau of Health Information in Australia reported in the quarter from January to March of 2023 the percentage of acute mental health episodes of care with at least one seclusion event in New South Wales was down in percentage points compared with the same quarter the previous year.[29]

Restraints

To restrain is to limit, restrict, or keep under control through deprivation or limitation of liberty and confinement. Restraints include both physical and chemical forms in the medical profession. Chemical restraints are defined as the involuntary emergency utilization of medications to control or subdue patients through sedation or restriction of movement. As needed, or PRN, medications are typically used in healthcare settings to manage clients' psychological processes and behaviors when they are experiencing mental conditions. Antipsychotics, antianxiety medications, and sedatives are standard medications used for this purpose in the medical field. No medications are approved by the Food and Drug Administration to be used as a chemical restraint in the United States.[30]

Physical restraints are any manual method, physical or mechanical device, material, or equipment that immobilizes or reduces the ability of a patient to move his or her arms, legs, body or head freely. There are wrist, ankle, and waist restraints. History reveals frequent utilization of camisoles or straitjackets to control psychiatric patients. And five-point-leather restraints were commonly used interventions to detain mental health patients in the 1980s and 1990s.

The implementation and continuation of staff educational processes on the topic of seclusion and restraints have reduced the hours of seclusion and restraint utilization in most psychiatric settings. The Substance Abuse and Mental Health Services Administration (SAMHSA) study in 2018 revealed that 84% to 91% of the sampled facilities using seclusion and restraints had reduction strategies implemented.[31] Reduction interventional strategies suggested by the Mental Health Commission include leadership, engagement, education, data, debriefing, environment, regulation, and staffing. Included in the mandated Health and Human Services educational processes is training on alternative methods for handling behaviors, symptoms, and situations that have been traditionally managed through the utilization of seclusion and restraints within psychiatric institutions. Data collected by CMS in 2015 and 2020 revealed a reduction in restraint utilization by 220,615 hours (2015–443,956 hours; 2020–223,341 hours) in U.S. psychiatric settings.[32] The utilization of restraints in psychiatric hospitals is exhibited in Figure 1.12.

A 2020 analysis in Austria and Switzerland that included a total of 29,477 patients hospitalized in 140 hospitals revealed the prevalence rate for the use of at least one

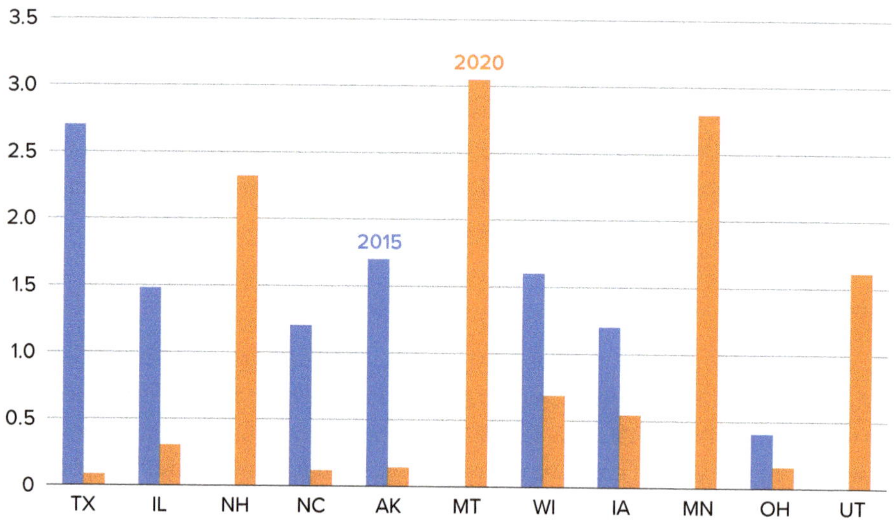

FIGURE 1.12 Restraint Episodes 2015 and 2020 (Overall Rate per 1000)[33]

restraint over a 30-day period was 8.7%, with mechanical restraints representing the highest proportion of restraint types used (55.0%). The main reason for restraint use was fall prevention (43.8%), followed by confusion or delirious behavior (20.4%).[34] The Bureau of Health Information in Australia reported in the January to March of 2023 quarter that the percentage of acute mental health episodes of care with at least one physical restraint event in New South Wales was up a few percentage points compared with the same quarter the previous year.[35]

Even with educational processes initiated in the 1990s, problems with seclusion and restraints are still prevalent, as illustrated in Box 1.1. Over the years, there have been many different treatment modalities used with psychiatric patients. Some of which, in this current time, are considered to be barbaric in nature. Examining the medical procedures of the past and present can assist in understanding the evolution of diagnosis, treatment, and prognosis encompassing individuals experiencing psychiatric illnesses.

BOX 1.1 North Carolina State Hospital

In March of 2004, the U.S. Department of Justice released the findings of their investigation of all four of North Carolina's state hospitals, which included inappropriate use of restraints and seclusion and failure to ensure reasonable safety of patients. It cited several instances of patients being on combinations or high doses of psychotropic medications in the absence of any justification for utilization in their records. It also reported that nearly half of all North Carolina state hospital patients have a regular or PRN order for benzodiazepines but no justification for such utilization in the patients' charts: "This practice constitutes chemical restraint, which is in violation of federal regulations ... and does not conform to generally accepted professional standards."[36]

Noninvasive Treatment Modalities

Malarial Therapy

Developed by an Austrian psychiatrist in 1917, the treatment modality of malarial therapy was used to treat neurosyphilis. Patients were given the malarial parasite to induce malarial fever, and supporting documentation exhibits that the majority of clients became well, demonstrated signs of improvement, or the progression of the mental disease process was eradicated. This procedure initiated the onset of many other treatment modalities for psychiatric conditions during the early 20th century. The major mental illness receiving the progression of diverse treatment modalities was "dementia praecox," currently known as schizophrenia.

Barbiturate Induced Deep Sleep Therapy

This treatment modality was founded in 1915 by an Italian psychiatrist and was popularized in 1920 by a Swiss psychiatrist for the treatment of schizophrenia. It was used primarily on clients who were manic or very agitated. Sodium Amytal was the main drug used to induce a 7- to 14-day period of deep narcosis for patients, and bronchopneumonia was a recurrent complication from the treatment modality.

Deep sleep therapy (DST) was notably combined with electroconvulsive shock therapy and other treatment modalities to promote toleration of the electroconvulsive shock therapy procedures and eradicate client memory development of the procedures being performed on them during the 1950s and 1960s in the United Kingdom and Canada. During the 1960s to 1970s, 24 clients expired in an Australian hospital from the utilization of DST. In 1993, the High Court upheld a permanent stay on legal proceedings against the doctors, granting them immunity against prosecution.[37]

Insulin Shock

The insulin shock procedure originated in Berlin, developed in 1927 by a Viennese physician practicing in one of their hospitals. In 1933, the physician made his discovery public. A Polish Austrian psychiatrist then introduced insulin shock therapy to the psychiatric community in the year 1933; the treatment modality was commonly used in the United States during the 1940s and 1950s.

Schizophrenic clients were injected with large amounts of insulin (100–450 units), inducing epileptic seizures, with subsequent onset of a coma that was allowed to last for approximately an hour; IV glucose was then used to terminate the coma. Research demonstrates that some schizophrenic conditions would improve after 30 to 40 treatments of insulin-induced shock. The risks involved with insulin shock therapy involved brain damage and death; one case study demonstrated a 1% to 10% mortality rate with the procedure.[38] When antipsychotic medications became obtainable, the procedure utilization declined and was finally eradicated in the mid-1960s.

Cardiazol Shock Therapy

Also known as Metrazol, the shock therapy procedure was developed in 1934 by a Hungarian neuropathologist/psychiatrist, and the medication replaced insulin shock therapy in some countries. It was believed during this time frame that there was a link between schizophrenia and epilepsy, and inducing tonic-clonic seizures in schizophrenic patients could elicit a cure for the mental illness.

The treatment modality proved most successful in clients diagnosed with depression. Cardiazol® (a cardiac stimulant) was administered at ten times the normal dosage in these treatment procedures to induce seizures in clients diagnosed with severe depression. A case study in 1939 demonstrated that 100% of the clients obtained full remission of their mood disorder.[39] The major controversy surrounding this treatment modality utilization was the trauma experienced by clients during the induced seizures, including joint dislocations, bone fractures, vertebral fractures, broken or loosened teeth, and bruises.

Electroconvulsive Therapy

Electroconvulsive therapy (ECT) was formulated by an Italian neurologist, and its use on clients began between the years 1937 to 1938. The exact mechanism for producing positive effects with the procedure is unknown, but seizures are electrically induced to obtain therapeutic effects with psychiatric illnesses, such as depression, mania, and catatonia. It is believed by some scientists that induced convulsions stimulate neurotransmitters in the brain, potentially producing feelings of euphoria.

The procedure is still used today, and the majority of clients who receive this modality of treatment are women suffering from severe depression. Diagnostic case studies have proven that ECT, as a treatment modality isolated by itself, is not effective for the treatment of mental conditions over prolonged periods of time. A major side effect of the procedure can be long-term memory loss, with past research data substantiating that up to 55% of clients receiving ECT were inflicted with permanent memory deficits.[40]

Current ECT procedural processes are argued to be less debilitating, with less permanent memory loss occurring in clients. Some studies have demonstrated that electroconvulsive therapy does not produce any anatomical structural damage in the human brain, but not all scientists agree with this conclusion, and those scientists argue that the ECT procedure generates hemorrhaging and destruction of neurons in the brain.

In the 1930s, electrodes were placed on both sides of the client's head, and 70–150 volts of electricity were administered over a 0.1–0.5 second time frame; clients typically received 6 to 12 ECT treatments. The current devices used for ECT treatment emit a brief-pulse current; this type of current will generate fewer side effects for psychiatric clients, and electrode placement is unilateral (only on the right side of the head), leaving the language and auditory memory centers in the left side of the brain unaffected by electrical currents. Figure 1.13 illustrates a 1945 ECT machine.

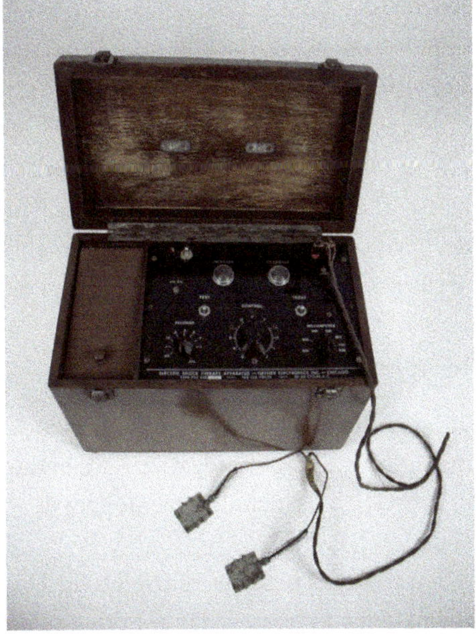

FIGURE 1.13 1945 Electric Shock Therapy Apparatus, Offner Electronics. Nebraska State Historical Society

These devices are classified by the Food and Drug Administration (FDA) as Class III devices, which are the highest risk class of medical devices in the nation. In 2018, the FDA reclassified uses for ECT devices (with special controls) into Class II for the treatment of catatonia or severe major depressive episodes associated with major depressive disorder or bipolar disorder in patients aged 13 years and older who are treatment resistant or who require rapid response treatment owing to the severity of their condition.[41]

United States

An American study in 2014 revealed that of the 969,277 patients with a mood disorder, 2,471 (0.25%) received ECT.[42] It is estimated that today, as many as 100,000 people in the United States receive ECT each year.[43] A 2019 analysis of three states (California, Vermont, and Illinois) revealed 62,602 patients received ECT, with women representing 62.3% of the patients.[44]

Other Countries

A 2014 study of European countries revealed that Slovakia and the Czech Republic offered ECT in 92% and 67% of their psychiatric facilities, with a 2.92 and 1.36 per 10,000 population utilization rate, respectively; Estonia offered ECT in less than 50% of their mental facilities and had an above 2 per 10,000 population utilization rate; Hungary, Lithuania, and Spain demonstrated medium ECT utilization in 50% of their psychiatric facilities, demonstrating rates with figures between 2 and 0.2 per 10,000 population; 43% of Poland's psychiatric facilities offer ECT; low accessibility to ECT is found in the Ukraine, Croatia, and Serbia, and Slovenia has banned ECT since 1994.[45]

It is estimated that approximately 75,000 ECT treatments are administered annually in Canada, with 90% of the treatments being administered on an outpatient basis.[46] Plus, in 2021, an analysis of ECT in England revealed there had been a gradual decline in utilization, with approximately 2,500 people per year receiving ECT; most of the patients were women (67%) and over 60 years of age (58%).[47]

Hydrotherapy

This treatment modality emerged in the 20th century and was used in cases of insomnia, agitation, suicidal ideation, and manic-depressive psychosis. The different types of hydrotherapy included needle sprays, sitz baths, continuous baths, showers, packs, and scotch douches.

Continuous baths were used to induce calming effects with clients; immersing the patients in fresh water at body temperature that lasted for hours or even days. Cold water packs at a temperature of 48–70 degrees Fahrenheit were used with clients for hours at a time; the patients were wrapped in the blanket packs from head to foot; agitated or excited clients could then rest, according to the logic of thinking during this time frame. The showers, needle sprays, and scotch douches were used on standing patients and consisted of sprays of water ejected at the clients, either hot or cold, or alternating both temperatures.

Invasive Treatment Modalities

Sterilization

Eugenics is a science that encompasses the improvement of hereditary qualities, usually in human beings (as by selective breeding). Mandatory sterilization laws were enacted in 1907 in the United States; these laws included both mentally retarded and mentally ill human beings for the compulsory sterilization procedure. The laws were incorporated through a then-held belief system of motivational factors surrounding eugenics, therapeutics, and punishment of individuals in society. It is estimated that approximately 65,000 individuals were mandatorily sterilized in the United States during the laws existence.[48]

In the state of Nebraska, mandatory sterilizations began in 1917, with a total of 902 individuals forced to undergo the medical procedure. It is documented that 80% of the individuals sterilized were categorized as "mentally deficient." The Beatrice State Developmental Center in Beatrice, Nebraska, which Nebraska referred to as the "Institution for Feebleminded Youth" in 1885, provided 752 of their patients for the mandatory sterilization procedures.[49] Ingleside or the HRC offered up 32 of their patients for mandatory sterilizations during the law's existence.[50]

Eugenics was practiced in Canada; the Sexual Sterilization Act (Alberta) from 1928 to 1972 created a eugenics board that could authorize the procedure; over 2,800 individuals were sterilized under this legislation.[51] And under the Sexual Sterilization Act (British Columbia), from 1933 to 1973, approximately 200 to 400 individuals were sterilized.[52]

In Sweden, from 1935 to 1976, under the Sterilization Act, there were approximately 63,000 people sterilized.[53] Germany enacted the "Racial Hygiene" law in 1934 with an initial 64,000 sterilizations approved by the Hereditary Health Courts. It is estimated that between 1934 and 1944, German doctors sterilized at least 400,000 individuals.[54]

Psychosurgery

Psychosurgery is defined as neurosurgery for mental diseases. The neurosurgical treatment consists of ablation or disconnection of brain tissue with the intent of changing affective or cognition states caused by mental disease. Today, psychosurgery is not commonly practiced.

Frontal Lobotomies

The leucotomy surgical procedure consists of two different operating standards: the prefrontal lobotomy and the transorbital lobotomy. Both procedures involve severing the frontal lobe of the human brain in psychiatric clients with surgical knives or ice picks to eradicate aggressive behaviors. Clients typically were reduced to an infant stage of functionality and had to be retrained in basic activities of daily living. Adverse effects of psychosurgery included a reduced capacity to learn and an inability to deal with experiences that required a fast reaction for planning.

A standard prefrontal lobotomy involves removing or damaging a small portion of the brain's frontal lobe in psychiatric clients and was developed in 1935 by a Portuguese neurologist. The procedure was typically performed on clients with obsessive disorders, severe depression, and schizophrenia.

The transorbital lobotomy, known as the Freeman-Watts procedure, did not have to be performed in a surgical room and took approximately 15 minutes to complete the operation. An ice pick (orbitoclast) was inserted through the orbit above the eyeball and was used to sever brain tissue in psychiatric clients. In the United States and Europe, between 1936 and 1956, approximately 60,000 individuals were lobotomized.[55]

Trepanation

The procedure of trepanation was one of the earliest modalities used in psychiatric cases. Ancient cultures believed that psychological conditions were generated by demons being trapped in a human being's skull. Trepanation, the process of drilling a hole in the skull, allowed the demons to escape from the human body, thus curing "insanity." The treatment modality was widely practiced until the early 20th century, then abandoned when other procedures were developed and implemented in the field of psychiatry. More than 1,500 trephined skulls have been uncovered throughout the world; from Europe, Scandinavia to North America, Russia, and China to South America.[56] Many of these past invasive and noninvasive treatment modalities were abandoned once psychopharmacology and psychotherapy were widely available.

Pharmacology

Paraldehyde was one of the first medications used for psychiatric conditions, and initial administration to patients occurred around the year 1882. The medication was found to be a safe hypnotic/sedative drug and was used in mental hospitals until the beginning of the 1950s. Barbital was first synthesized in 1902, with phenobarbital marketed and used as a popular sedative/hypnotic for clients, initiated in the year 1912.

The first antipsychotic drug, Thorazine (Chlorpromazine), was synthesized in France in 1950 and was recognized by a French psychiatrist as being effective with psychosis in 1952. Thorazine improved the quality of life for consumers through the alleviation of mental disease symptoms, including hallucinations, thought disorders, agitation, and delusions. The medication was "coined" by some psychiatrists as the "chemical lobotomy" because of the permanent adverse effects suffered by psychiatric clients, indicating brain damage occurrence with the medication's utilization.[57] In the 1990s, other psychotropic medications, such as Clozaril®, Risperdal®, Serdolect®, and Zypreza®, became available on the market that produced less debilitating side effects.

Reserpine was attributed to being effective with psychiatric disorders by an American psychiatrist in 1954. Reserpine blocks the vesicular transporter for neurotransmitters in the human brain, thus depleting synaptic connections and inducing stabilization of some psychiatric conditions. The medication is no longer used on the market due to its antihypertensive effects and adverse cholinergic side effects.

Lithium carbonate's mood stabilizing effect with bipolar disorder was discovered in 1948 but was banned in the United States until the 1970s. The medication is used to treat the manic phase in manic/depressive disorder by disrupting the transport processes of messages carried to neurons in the human brain.

The development of antidepressants improved the treatment outcomes for individuals diagnosed with depression. A medication called Marsalid® was used in 1958 for tuberculosis patients and was found to have antidepressant effects, but was replaced by Marplan®, Nardil®, and Parnate® due to its hepatotoxic effects. Currently, there are over 52 different antidepressant medications on the market.

In 1956, Congress approved $12 million to be allotted for the research surrounding clinical aspects of psychopharmacology, encompassing mental illness in the United States. Positive research outcomes with the utilization of psychopharmacology led to a decrease in client populations within mental institutions.

Psychotherapy

The term was first used in the 1890s to describe a technique of counseling that assists individuals with overcoming stress, emotional and relationship problems, and habits that interfere with everyday life skills. Psychotherapy can typically be referred to as "talk therapy" and is implemented to increase an individual's sense of well-being and capacity for self-observation. The techniques used in psychotherapy are centered around relationship building, dialogue, communication, and behavioral changes. Psychotherapy encompasses several subsystems, including psychoanalytic, behavioral, humanistic, cognitive, and systemic therapy avenues that can be used when assisting clients in the psychiatric profession. Psychotherapy can also be categorized into individual, group, family, cognitive dialectical behavioral, interpersonal, and eye movement desensitization and reprocessing therapies.

Psychoanalysis, a form of psychotherapy, was developed by Sigmund Freud in the 1890s to assist clients afflicted with neurosis and hysteria. Dr. Freud focused on cases of a psychological nature that displayed no organic causative factors and argued that the psychological symptomatology was generated by childhood experiences that affected the unconscious mind. This treatment modality became very popular during the postwar era. Currently, there are over 32 institutions or centers in the United States that provide psychoanalytic training or treatment.

At present, many psychiatric hospitals and units in general hospitals have unblemished histories; they provide humane and effective treatment modalities and safe and therapeutic environments for their clients. A 2020 ranking of psychiatric hospitals listed Johns Hopkins Hospital in Baltimore, Maryland, first; McLean Hospital in Belmont, Massachusetts, second; Massachusetts General Hospital in Boston, third; and New York-Presbyterian University Hospital of Columbia and Cornell, fourth.[58] The global trend of closing state psychiatric hospitals and moving toward community-based mental health treatment is ongoing. There are positive and negative qualities to this process, and we need to understand the potential impacts on clients, families, and communities to obtain systematic mental healthcare delivery systems that are effective for society as a whole in low-, middle-, and high-income countries.

BOX 1.2 A Critical Thinking Synopsis—Do You Agree?

The institutionalization of many individuals who experienced mental conditions was practiced for centuries worldwide; this chapter serves as a building block for further exploration into the mental healthcare services continuum and lends insight into "why" changes in the provision of services in this branch of medicine evolved. The author of this book supports the global deinstitutionalization process, reduction of restraint and seclusion utilization, eradication of chemical restraints, and further development of mental health services that promote quality of life.

Main Points

1. Involuntary admissions (civil commitments) to psychiatric hospitals in the United States were common practice in the 19th century.
2. The majority of state psychiatric hospitals were originally built under the "Kirkbride Plan," which was formulated by Dr. Thomas Story Kirkbride through his 1845 book, *On the Construction, Organization, and General Arrangements of Hospitals for the Insane.*
3. After release from a psychiatric hospital in 1908, Mr. Beers wrote and published his book, *A Mind That Found Itself.* The book led to mental health care reform in the United States and other countries, instituting the National

Committee for Mental Hygiene in 1909, currently called the National Mental Health Association.

4. The World Health Organization launched a training program, "Strategies to End Seclusion and Restraints," in 2019. The organization acknowledges that seclusion and restraints, which generate physical and mental harm to patients, are widely prevalent practices in mental health care worldwide.
5. Over the years, there have been many different treatment modalities used with psychiatric patients, some of which, in this current time, are considered to be barbaric in nature.
6. Currently, many psychiatric hospitals and units in general hospitals have unblemished histories; they provide humane and effective treatment modalities and safe and therapeutic environments for their clients.

Notes

1. Substance Abuse and Mental Health Services Administration (2019), Civil Commitment and the Mental Health Care Continuum: Historical Trends and Principles for Law and Practice, https://www.samhsa.gov/resource/ebp/civil-commitment-mental-healthcare-continuum-historical-trends-principles-law (accessed December 12, 2021), 1–43. pp. 3.
2. National Institute of Mental Health (2020), New NIMH Strategic Plan Paves the Way for Advances in Mental Health Research, https://www.nimh.nih.gov/news/science-news/2020/new-nimh-strategic-plan-paves-the-way-fpr-advances-in-mental-health (accessed December 11, 2021).
3. Sorbo, Emanuela (2016), Ruins of Memory: A Sustainable Conservation for the Material and Immaterial Values of the Former Psychiatric Hospitals in Italy, https://doi:10.1016/proeng.2016.08.815 (accessed December 11, 2021).
4. Appleton, V.E. (1967), *Psychiatry in Canada a Century Ago, Canadian Psychiatric Association Journal,* 12(4), https://www.journals.sagepub.com/doi/abs/10.117/070674376701200402 (accessed December 11, 2021), pp. 345–361.
5. Jeanroy, Aurora (2020), Mental Health Laws in France: A Historical View, European Community Based Mental Health Service Providers, https://www.eucoms.net/wp-content/uploads/2020/01/Laws-the-French-context-Aurora-Jeanroy-pdf (accessed December 11, 2021).
6. Curwen, John, MD, et al. (1885), *Memoir of Thomas S. Kirkbride MD, LLD,* Prepared by Direction of the Associates of Medical Superintendents of American Institution for the Insane, Warren PA: E. Rowan & Co, pp. 35–37.
7. Curwen, John, MD, et al. (1885), *Memoir of Thomas S. Kirkbride MD, LLD,* prepared by direction of the Associates of Medical Superintendents of American Institution for the Insane, Warren PA: E. Rowan & Co, pp. 35–37.
8. Eastern State Hospital, America's first psychiatric hospital since 1773, http://www.esh.dmhmrsas.virginia.gov/Mission.html (accessed May 20, 2019), pp. 1–2.
9. May 5, 1817: Founding of the Friends Asylum for the Relief of Persons Deprived of the Use of Their Reason, https://www.awb.com/dailydose/?p=1196. (accessed October 25, 2021).

10. Pilgrim State Hospital, abandoned photography at Opacity, http://www.opacity.us/site23_pilgrim_state_hospital.htm. (accessed May 6, 2018), pp. 1–2.
11. Pilgrim State Hospital, abandoned photography at Opacity, http://www.opacity.us/site23_pilgrim_state_hospital.htm (accessed May 6, 2018), pp. 1–2.
12. Harvard Medical School (2021), McLean Hospital: About McLean, https://hms.harvard.edu/affiliates/mcclean-hospital (accessed April 19, 2021).
13. Adams County Historical Society, Hastings State Hospital, http://www.rootsweb.ancestry.com/-asylums/hastings_nb/index.html (accessed November 16, 2017).
14. Adams County Historical Society, Hastings State Hospital, http://www.rootsweb.ancestry.com/-asylums/hastings_nb/index.html (accessed November 16, 2017).
15. State of California (2021), California Department of State Hospitals-Napa, https://www.dsh.ca.gov/napa (accessed April 19, 2021).
16. Makeenko, Viktoriia (2020), Mombello Psychiatric Hospital, abandoned spaces, https://www.abandonedspaces.com/hospital//mombello-psychiatric-hospital.html?edg-c=1 (accessed December 6, 2021).
17. Tiao, Janice (2016), The history of Bethlem Hospital, Hektoen International, https://www.hekint.org/2017/02/22/the-history-of-bethlem-hospital (accessed December 6, 2021).
18. Rossiter, Kate, Dr., and Clarkson, Annalise (2013), Opening Ontario's "saddest chapter: A social history of Huronia Regional Centre, Canadian Journal of Disability Studies, 2(3), https://doi.org/10.15353/cjds.v2i3.99 (accessed December 6, 2021), pp.1–30.
19. Asylum Projects (2021), Charenton, https://www.asylumprojects.org/index.php.title=charenton (accessed December 6, 2021).
20. The Extra Mile-Points of Light Volunteer Pathway, Clifford W. Beers, http://www.extramile.us/honorees/beers.cfm (accessed May 20, 2020), pp.1–2.
21. The Extra Mile-Points of Light Volunteer Pathway, Clifford W. Beers, https://www.extramile.us/honorees/beers.cfm (accessed May 20, 2020), pp.1–2.
22. Wagner, Steve (2012), State hospitals are still snake pits of patient abuse, betrayal of the public. Psychiatric Crime Database, https://www.psychcrime.org/articles/index.php?vd=12 (accessed February 6, 2020).
23. Department of Health and Human Services, National Mental Health Services Survey (N-MHSS): 2018 data on mental health treatment facilities, Substance Abuse and Mental Health Services Administration, https://www.samhsa.gov/data/report/National-Mental-Health-Services-Survey-N-MHSS-2018- Data-on-Mental-Health-Treatment-Facilities (accessed April 24, 2021).
24. Lepping, Peter, et al. (2016), Comparison of restraint data from four countries, *Soc Psychiatry Psychiatr Epidemiol,* 51(9):1301–1309, https://doi:10.1007/s00127-016-1203-x, https://www.pubmed.ncbi.nlm.nih.gov/27147243 (accessed December 11, 2021).
25. Knox, Daryl, M.D., et al. (2012), Use and avoidance of seclusion and restraint: Consensus Statement of the American Association for Emergency Psychiatry Project BETA Seclusion and Restraint Workgroup, *Western Journal of Emergency Medicine,* 13(1) https://pubmed.ncbi.nlm.nih.gov/22461919/ (accessed December 11, 2021), pp. 35–40.
26. Alhaj, Hamid, MD, PhD (2019), A practical guide to the use of seclusion in mental health settings, National Association of Psychiatric Intensive Care, MCCPsych, https://napicu.

org.uk/wo-content/uploads/2019/04/HAMID-BAP-NAPICU-Cambridge (accessed October 23, 2021).

27. Medicare Hospital Compare (2015 & 2020), Inpatient psychiatric facility reporting program, quality measure data by state, https://www.medicare.gov (accessed December 6, 2020).

28. Medicare Hospital Compare (2015 & 2020), Inpatient psychiatric facility reporting program, quality measure data by state, https://www.medicare.gov (accessed December 6, 2020).

29. Bureau of Health Information (2023), Seclusion and restraint supplement, January to March 2023, https://www.bhi.nsw.gov.au/data/assets/pdf_file/0010/888139/BHI_HQ52_JAN-MAR_2023_SECLUSION_AND_RESTRAINT_SUPP.pdf#:~:text= Percentage%20of%20acute%20mental%20health%20episodes%20of%20care,restraint%20event%2095.4%25%20with%20no%20physical%20restraint%20event (accessed, August 16, 2023).

30. Kincaid, Linda, MPH, and Tomasso, Vanessa, BS (2013), Chemical restraint: Elder abuse in long-term care, California Advocates for Nursing Home Reform, https://www.napsa.now.org/wp-content/uploads/2013/10/NAPSA-chemicalrestraints.pdf (accessed February 6, 2020).

31. Department of Health and Human Services, National Mental Health Services Survey (N-MHSS): 2018 data on mental health treatment facilities, Substance Abuse and Mental Health Services Administration, https://www.samhsa.gov/data/report/ National-Mental-Health-Services-Survey-N-MHSS-2018- Data-on-Mental-Health-Treatment-Facilities (accessed April 24, 2021).

32. Medicare Hospital Compare (2015 & 2020), Inpatient psychiatric facility reporting program, quality measure data by state, https://www.medicare.gov (accessed December 6, 2020)

33. Medicare Hospital Compare (2015 & 2020), Inpatient psychiatric facility reporting program, quality measure data by state, https://www.medicare.gov (accessed December 6, 2020).

34. Thomann, Silvia, et al. (2020), Restraint use in the acute care hospital setting: a cross-sectional multi-centre study, *Int J Nurs Stud*, 114:103807, https://pubmed.ncbi.nlm.nih.gov/33217663/ (accessed August 16, 2023).

35. Bureau of Health Information (2023), Seclusion and restraint supplement, January to March 2023, https://www.bhi.nsw.gov.au/data/assets/pdf_file/0010/888139/BHI_HQ52_JAN-MAR_2023_SECLUSION_AND_RESTRAINT_SUPP.pdf#:~:text= Percentage%20of%20acute%20mental%20health%20episodes%20of%20care,restraint%20event%2095.4%25%20with%20no%20physical%20restraint%20event (accessed, August 16, 2023).

36. Wagner, Steve (2012), State hospitals are still snake pits of patient abuse, betrayal of the public. Psychiatric Crime Database, https://www.psychcrime.org/articles/index.php?vd=12 (accessed February 6, 2020).

37. Sainty, Lane (2018), Two doctors connected to the "deep sleep therapy" medical scandal are suing over an ABC journalist's Scientology book, https://www.buzzfeed.com/lanesainty/two-doctors-connected-to-the-deep-sleep-therapy-medical (accessed October 26, 2021).

38. American experience, primary sources: Insulin coma therapy, https://www.pbs.com/f/insulin+com+therapy.doc (accessed February 6, 2020).

39. Kragh, Jesper, PhD (2010), Shock therapy in Danish psychiatry, Institute of Public Health, University of Copenhagen, Medical History, 54(3). https://doi:10.1017/s0025727300004646, https://europemc.org/aricle/MED/20592884 (accessed December 5, 2020), pp. 341–364.

40. MacQueen, Glenda, PhD et al. (2007), The long-term impact of treatment with electroconvulsive therapy on discrete memory systems in patients with bipolar disorder, *Journal of Psychiatry and Neuroscience,* 32(4), https://www.ncbi.nlm.nih.gov/pmc/articles/PMC1911194/ (accessed December 5, 2020), pp. 241–249.

41. Walsh, Sandy (2018), FDA in brief: FDA takes action to ensure regulation of electroconvulsive therapy devices better protects patients, reflects current understanding of safety and effectiveness, U.S Department of Health and Human Services, Food and Drug Administration, Center for Devices and Radiological, https://www.fda.gov/news-events/fda-brief/fda-brief-fda-takes-action-to-ensure-regulation-of-electroconvulsive-therapy-devices (accessed April 25, 2021).

42. Wilkinson, Samuel, MD, et al. (2018), Identifying recipients of electroconvulsive therapy: Data from privately insured Americans, *Psyciatr Serv,* 69(5). https://doi:10.1176/appi.ps.201700364, https://www.ncbi.nlm.nih.gov/29385954 (accessed December 12, 2021), pp. 542–548.

43. Windmoor Healthcare (2023), Electroconvulsive therapy, https://windmoor.com/treatment-services/outpatient-treatment/electroconvulsive-therapy/ (accessed August 16, 2023).

44. Luccarelli, James, MD., et al. (2021), Demographics of patients receiving electroconvulsive therapy based on state-mandated reporting data, *J ECT,* 36 (4), https://www.ncbi.nlm.nih/gov/pmc/articles/PMC7677170/ (accessed August 16, 2023), pp. 229–233.

45. Gazdag, Gabor, et al. (2017), *Use of electroconvulsive therapy in central-eastern European countries: An overview, Psychiatria Danubina,* 29(2), https://pubmed.ncbi.nlm.nih.gov/28636570/ (accessed December 12, 2021), pp. 136–140. pp. 138.

46. Canadian Agency for Drugs and Technologies in Health (2014), Delivery of electroconvulsive therapy in non-hospital settings: A review of the safety and guidelines, https://www.ncbi.nlm.nih.gov/25520991 (accessed December 12, 2021).

47. The British Psychological Society (2021), *A second independent audit of electroconvulsive therapy in England, 2019: usage, demographics, consent, and adherence to guidelines and legislation, psychology and psychotherapy: Theory, research, and practice,* 94(3), https://doi.org/10.1111/papt.12335 (accessed January 5, 2022), pp. 603–619.

48. Kaelber, Lutz, Associate Professor of Sociology (2012), Eugenics: Compulsory sterilization in 50 American states, University of Vermont, https://www.uvm.edu/-lkaelber/eugenics/ (accessed April 25, 2021).

49. Kaelber, Lutz, Associate Professor of Sociology (2012), Nebraska eugenics, University of Vermont, https://www.uvm.edu/lkaelber/eugenics/NE/NE.html (accessed April 25, 2021).

50. Kaelber, Lutz, Associate Professor of Sociology (2012), Nebraska eugenics, University of Vermont, https://www.uvm.edu/lkaelber/eugenics/NE/NE.html (accessed April 25, 2021).

51. de Bruin, Tabitha and Robertson, Gerald (2019), Eugenics in Canada, *The Canadian Encyclopedia,* https://www. thecanadianencyclopedia.ca/en/article/eugenics (accessed December 12, 2021).

52. de Bruin, Tabitha and Robertson, Gerald (2019), Eugenics in Canada, *The Canadian Encyclopedia*, https://www. thecanadianencyclopedia.ca/en/article/eugenics (accessed December 12, 2021).

53. Shaw, Laura and Kurbegovic, Erna (2014), Sweden, https://www.eugenicsarchive.ca/discover/tree/51c27497b894oa54000009 (accessed December 12, 2021).

54. Reilly, Philip (2015), "Eugenics and involuntary sterilization: 1907–2015," 16, 351–368, https://doi.org/10.1146/annurevgenom-090314-024930 (accessed December 12, 2021).

55. Faria, Miguel, Jr. (2013), Violence, mental illness, and the brain—a brief history of psychosurgery: Part I—from trephination to lobotomy, *Surgical Neurology International*, 4:49, https://doi:10.4103/2152-7806.110146, https://pubmed.ncbi.nlm.nih.gov/23646259 (accessed December 12, 2021).

56. Faria, Miguel (2015), Neolithic trepanation decoded—a unifying hypothesis: Has the mystery as to why primitive surgeons performed cranial surgery been solved? *Surg Neurol Int*, 6:72. https://doi:10.4103/2152-7806.156634, https://ncbi.nlm.nih.gov/25984386 (accessed December 12, 2021).

57. Citizens Commission on Human Rights (2011), Thorazine: Chemical lobotomy? http://www.cchr.florida.org/thorazine-chemical-lobotomy (accessed May 5, 2018).

58. U.S. News and World Report (2020), Best hospitals for psychiatry, New York, NY, www.health.usnews.com/best-hospitals/rankings/psychiatry (accessed April 19, 2021).

Credits

Fig. 1.11: Data Source: Medicare.gov.

Fig. 1.12: Data Source: Medicare.gov.

Fig. 1.13: Nebraska State Historical Society Library/Archives, "ECT machine." Copyright © by History Nebraska. Reprinted with permission.

CHAPTER 2

Deinstitutionalization and Transinstitutionalization

The main objective of this chapter is for the reader to have an increased understanding of the deinstitutionalization and transinstitutionalization processes within the mental health care continuum globally and the influential factors of each operation.

Deinstitutionalization, which began in 1955, is explained as the discharging of patients from psychiatric hospitals and the subsequent partial or full closure of the institutions. It has been identified that there are essentially three major reasons for this global process occurring:

1. Money
2. New psychotropic medications available
3. Poorly perceived reputations of the institutions

The process of deinstitutionalization has varied from country to country and from state to state. Many individuals believe that deinstitutionalization "humanizes" mental health services. This chapter explores the worldwide deinstitutionalization process that is still occurring in many countries, the aspects of transinstitutionalization, and the positive attributes that are connected to global deinstitutionalization.

Perceptions on the reason base for mental health decline have evolved over the centuries; today, we now know that there are multifactorial dynamics involved that can include genetics, environment, childhood trauma, substance misuse, brain chemistry, and stressful events. In the past (1864 to 1889), the West Virginia Psychiatric Hospital (Trans-Allegheny Lunatic Asylum) compiled a list of reasons or believed causes of insanity, including the following:

- Novel reading
- Laziness
- Egotism
- Asthma
- Imaginary female trouble

- Female disease
- Mental excitement
- Jealousy
- Greediness
- Bad habits
- Fighting fire
- The war
- Immoral life[1]

The following 2.1 document is a submission to the Governor of Nebraska in 1906 containing the potential causes of insanity.

DOCUMENT 2.1 1906 Report, "State Hospital Insane." Nebraska Literary Commission. The Atrium, 1200 N. Street, Suite 120. Lincoln, Nebraska 68508-2023.

ALLEGED CAUSE OF INSANITY OF PATIENTS

Admitted during the Biennial Period ending November 30th, 1906.

	Males	Females	Totals
Alcoholism	22	0	22
Brain Fever	1	0	1
Business Reverses	1	0	1
Child Birth	0	1	1
Cerebro Spinal Meningitis	1	0	1
Arterio Sclerosis	1	0	1
Domestic Trouble	2	0	2
Epilepsy	12	2	14
Dissipation	3	0	3
Disappointment in love	1	0	1
Grief	1	0	1
Gambling	1	0	1
Hereditary	21	9	30
Injury and Measles	1	0	1
Injury	2	0	2
Injury to head	6	0	6
Imbecility	4	0	4

(continued)

	Males	Females	Totals
La Grippe	1	0	1
Masturbation	9	0	9
Morphine and Drugs	2	0	2
Overstudy	1	0	1
Paralysis	0	1	1
Spiritualism	1	0	1
Religion	4	0	4
Senility	14	3	17
Sunstroke	6	1	7
Syphilis	2	1	3
Typhoid Fever	1	0	1
Unknown	42	17	59
Totals	**163**	**35**	**198**

Deinstitutionalization in the United States

In the United States, the movement toward deinstitutionalization in the 1970s and 1980s is also partially attributed to the labor laws passed in the 1970s that mandated patients be paid minimum wages for the work they performed while housed in mental facilities. The passage of Medicaid in 1965 also offered more incentive for deinstitutionalization because the program excluded coverage for individuals in psychiatric institutions. Plus, the Ombudsman Reconciliation Act, passed in 1981, terminated the federal government's role in providing services to individuals experiencing mental illness. Between 1955 and 1994, there were roughly 487,000 patients with serious mental illness (SMI) released from state hospitals in the United States.[2] Document 2.2 reveals the age and diagnosis of clients admitted to a psychiatric hospital in 1906.

The main focus in the United States was the provision of community-based services, but the process in many states did not evolve in an efficient manner. It is suggested by many that poor planning and execution of the community-based process resulted in adverse consequences for many people experiencing mental illness. In New York State, the inpatient psychiatric bed count has dropped, yet the promise of better treatment at a lower cost has yet to be fulfilled.[3] By 1973, the number of patients in California's state mental hospitals dropped to 7,000, and in 2015, 55% of individuals experiencing chronic homelessness reported they had emotional or psychiatric conditions.[4]

It was estimated in 2004 that there were 100,000 psychiatric beds available in the United States. By 2010, the number dropped to 43,000 and to roughly 37,000

DOCUMENT 2.2 1906 Report "State Hospital for Insane." Nebraska Library Commission. The Atrium, 1200 North Street, Suite 120, Lincoln, Nebraska 68508-2023.

AGE OF PATIENTS WHEN ADJUDGED INSANE

Admitted during the Biennial Period ending November 30th, 1906.

Years—	Males	Females	Total
Between 15 to 25	16	6	22
Between 25 to 35	38	14	52
Between 35 to 45	32	2	34
Between 45 to 55	26	6	32
Between 55 to 65	22	4	26
Between 65 to 75	15	2	17
Between 75 to 85	12	0	12
Between 85 to 95	2	1	3
Totals	**163**	**35**	**198**
Average Age	**46**	**38**	**44**

FORMS OF DISEASE OF PATIENTS

Admitted during the Biennial Period ending November 30th, 1906.

Disease—	Males	Females	Totals
Acute Mania	4	0	4
Chronic Mania	11	2	13
Delusional Mania	42	0	42
Dementia	0	7	7
Dementia Atonica	1	0	1
Dementia Praecox	0	6	6
Epileptic	11	2	13
Epileptic Dementia	5	2	7
Epileptic Mania	3	0	3
Hysteria	0	1	1
Imbecility	8	3	11
Inebriate	2	0	2
Melancholia	2	7	9
Morphinism	1	0	1

(continued)

Disease—	Males	Females	Totals
Primary Dementia	2	0	2
Paresis	16	0	16
Paranoia	2	0	2
Senile Dementia	22	5	27
Secondary Dementia	29	0	29
Senile Epilepsy	2	0	2
Totals	**163**	**35**	**198**

beds in 2016, and currently, the number continues to drop.[5] As of 2020, there were 12,275 registered community mental health treatment facilities nationwide; 9,834 were less than 24-hour outpatient facilities, while 1,806 were 24-hour inpatient facilities.[6] Figure 2.1 portrays the number of psychiatric hospitals per country (the U.S. number is 195 facilities in 42 states). In 2019, it was estimated that only 44.8% of individuals experiencing a mental condition received treatment, and only 65.5% of individuals with an SMI received treatment in America.[7] According to Mental Health America, in 2022, over half (56%) of adults with a mental illness received no treatment, estimating that over 27 million individuals are going untreated.[8]

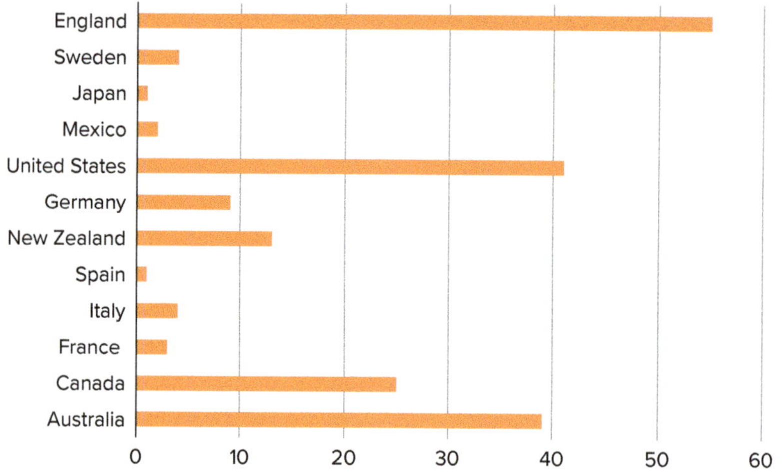

FIGURE 2.1 Number of Psychiatric Hospitals per Country[11]

Global Deinstitutionalization

A global study of 40 countries across all World Health Organization (WHO) regions in 2022 revealed a consensus that all countries should provide 30 to 60 psychiatric beds per 100,000/population.[9] Data identified that there were median psychiatric bed rates of 1.9/100,000 in low-income, 6.3/100,000 median in lower middle-income, median of 24.3/100,000 in upper middle-income, and 52.6/100,000 in high-income countries.[10]

France

Deinstitutionalization in France began with the process of sectorization, which is mental health services that have been organized in sectors, with each team providing care for 54,000 individuals. The process focuses on community-based treatment through community health centers, with hospitalization as needed. It is also highly focused on continuity of care between the two establishments. In 2018, France had decreased its hospital psychiatric care beds to 55,000 (from 100,000 in 1980).[12]

Italy

Italy is one of the forerunners in deinstitutionalization. Again, Basaglia Law (named after Italian psychiatrist Franco Basaglia) was instituted in 1978; it contained directives for closing all state-funded psychiatric hospitals in Italy. The country has moved toward community-based mental health care services with psychiatric units in general hospitals that contain a limited number of beds. In 2018, Italy had 5,358 psychiatric beds in its country.[13] It has been recognized by some mental health professionals that Trieste, Italy, is one of the most successful cities in the deinstitutionalization process because of the establishment of effective Community Mental Health Centers (CMHCs).

United Kingdom

In the United Kingdom, deinstitutionalization was initiated with the 1971 "Parliamentary White Paper" that was developed by the Department of Health. A policy was subsequently implemented known as Care in the Community that instituted the closure of all state psychiatric hospitals, which was obtained by 2015. The development of community-based mental healthcare centers and psychiatric units in general hospitals were established. Currently, there are 24,524 psychiatric beds available in the United Kingdom.[14]

Canada

Canada's deinstitutionalization process was initiated in the 1960s. It is estimated that the greatest amount of bed closures occurred between 1975 and 1981, with 62.2% of the beds removed from service.[15] In 2017, the federal government committed $5 billion over 10 years to support mental health services.[16] Canada continues to work on developing CMHCs and is establishing other venues for community psychiatric care services, such as telemedicine.

Spain

"Psychiatric reform" is the terminology used in Spain for deinstitutionalization. The process is partially successful in this country, with the reduction of 60% of their beds. But there has been retention of some psychiatric institutions for mental health care treatment versus closure. The establishment of community-based mental health services and the development of psychiatric units in general hospitals remains ongoing.

Germany

The movement toward community-based mental health services in Germany began in the 1970s. *The Care Quality Commission Report* recommended restructuring of mental health services and psychiatric hospitals. Currently, there are 274 psychiatric hospitals, 401 mental health units in general hospitals, and 63 mental health outpatient facilities in Germany.[17]

Positive Attributes of Deinstitutionalization

There have been many established positive aspects identified with the closing of state-funded psychiatric facilities. Obviously stated, for many clients, it led to a better quality of life through improved living conditions. Some studies also identified that there was an improvement in life skills for individuals while residing outside of mental institutions. There is also the promotion of human and civil rights, increased family involvement, improved focus on treatment, social inclusion, and a decreased potential for revictimization in community-based treatment versus institutionalization processes.

Promotion of Human and Civil Rights

All individuals in society have the right to receive health care (physical or mental) in the least restrictive environment. A least restrictive environment is considered to be a physical setting that places the least restraint on an individual's freedom of movement and independence in relation to their treatment needs. This also includes using the least intrusive treatment modalities for an individual's diagnosis. Plus, the least restrictive entails a person's liberty and autonomy; individuals have the right to make decisions about their lives and treatment. A community-based setting for mental health care reinforces an individual's human rights, whereas institutionalization is more restrictive.

Civil rights are personal rights guaranteed and protected by the U.S. Constitution and federal laws enacted by Congress. Civil rights encompass a wide spectrum of areas that protect people's physical and mental integrity, life, and safety, including the right to vote, to marry, to have children, to obtain education, to use public facilities, a right to privacy, a right to religion and a right to speech/expression. These laws were developed so all persons in the United States have a right to receive health care and human services in a nondiscriminatory manner.

Community inclusion involves living and finding meaningful roles in a community without discrimination. The ability to obtain community inclusion is a legal right that supports general medical, cognitive, and mental health and wellness. Promoting community inclusion for those in recovery from mental illness is a necessity to decrease stigmatization, isolation, and discrimination, thus, improving the quality of life for all individuals that reside within a community.

Increased Family Involvement

Having individuals recovering from mental illness in a community-based setting versus an institution allows for increased family involvement. Family support is important for the recovery process. Education in the family system is key for establishing healthy relationship interactions that focus on improving an individual's mental health versus the family problems contributing to the disorder or making it worse.

Family members providing encouragement and understanding during recovery assist in formulating acceptance. Families can also assist a family member experiencing a mental illness through encouragement of self-management, whether it involves medication compliance or other coping strategies. When a person's illness can be managed effectively or full recovery can be obtained, it enhances an overall sense of well-being and an individual's quality of life.

Mental illnesses can be considered family diseases, especially if based in abuse or substance misuse within the family system; in these instances, the family can contribute to the development of a mental condition. Focusing on the family structure dysfunction that contributes to mental health decline and providing education and therapy to all members of the family system would improve familial quality of life.

Focus on Treatment

The deinstitutionalization process allows for a focus on treatment rather than separating and isolating a person from society. Community inclusion by and through CMHCs allows for an integrated approach, with treatment, promotion, and prevention being equally important aspects. A high level of mental health is maintained in an environment that protects basic civil, human, socioeconomic, and cultural rights. Thus, the eradication of institutionalization for many experiencing mental conditions can be viewed as a healthier and more humane recovery process.

The recovery process varies for individuals and is a process of each individual establishing support and self-care techniques and treatments that work best in their particular situation; for some individuals, that can mean avoidance of people and situations that increase stress levels. Community-based housing can provide a less stressful environment for this process versus institutionalization to increase the potential for neuroplasticity and neurogenesis. There is a growing body of evidence that both the changing of neuron connections and the development of new neurons and glial cells can aid in recovery from mental illness. Facilitating an environment conducive to these recovery processes occurring is beneficial for mental health treatment.

Decreased Potential for Revictimization

Arguments encompassing retraumatization of patients by and through the psychiatric institution hospitalization process have been a topic of discussion for centuries. There are years of documented cases as evidence to substantiate that being victimized as a patient in a psychiatric hospital is based in reality. Patients can experience trauma by being the victim of staff or peer behaviors or by being exposed to adverse behaviors by other patients toward staff or other peers. Anger, aggression, and violence are often commonplace occurrences in these institutions. Crisis intervention teams are used to decrease the potential of harm with violent patient outbreaks, but there is no guarantee that injury/harm will not be sustained during violence exposure by other institutionalized patients.

Reviews on the prevalence of victimization within the mental healthcare system established that clients were exposed to other violent or frightening patients in 51.2% of the cases, 50% of the individuals experienced badgering or name calling by another patient, being committed against their own will occurred for 55.9% of the individuals, 40% reported experiencing theft, 7.1% reported being sexually assaulted by another patient and 3.5% by staff, and being physically assaulted by staff occurred in 10.6% of the cases.[18]

Aggression

A study in 2018 revealed that there were 157 security calls in a 6-month period for significant violent or aggressive behavior at a New York psychiatric unit.[19] A medication intervention was incorporated in the majority of these security calls. Another study conducted in 2011, which encompassed data from 11 countries, revealed that 32.4% of patients admitted to psychiatric facilities engaged in aggressive behavior or violence.[20] In 2021, an assessment of 146 studies concluded that the prevalence of aggressive behavior on psychiatric wards varied from 8% to 76%.[21] All the studies revealed that aggression and violence are common occurrences in psychiatric units throughout the world.

Sexual Abuse

There is also the potential for sexual violence to be conducted against patients, either by peers or employees in psychiatric institutions. In 2018, the United Kingdom Care Quality Commission revealed that there were 273 alleged sexual assaults in psychiatric facilities that were reported to the National Health Service during a 3-month period.[22] A 2012 survey of state hospital directors in the United States revealed that 7% of patients within the previous year had been victims of major sexual misconduct.[23] Another survey of facility directors revealed that over a 6-year period, 36% dealt with allegations of a staff member sexually assaulting a patient.[24] One major dilemma arises with these issues because the patients have a mental condition diagnosis. Many times, their reports of misconduct by staff are not taken seriously.

Coercion

Coercive measures in psychiatric institutions can lead to harm and, in some cases, death. Injuries during implementation and/or utilization of physical restraints were reported in 0.8%–4% of the cases.[25] Two studies revealed venous thrombosis embolism in restrained patients (38% and 11.6% of patients restrained) with prophylaxis treatment prescribed.[26] It was also identified that there were other forms of injuries/physical trauma reported in eight studies, including minor skin lesions, pressure sores, bruises, lacerations, contusions, fractures, and head injuries.[27]

Ending coercion in mental health care entails the reduction and elimination of coercive measures that are involuntary, forced, or nonconsensual practices. These practices can include restraints, seclusion, administration of sedative medications, constant observation, voluntary admissions being held against their will, inappropriate forced admissions, and providing any treatment without consent. The utilization of coercive practices can traumatize or retraumatize individuals, potentially generating adverse responses with regard to treatment and service providers. Thus decreasing the effectiveness of an individual's recovery process. The WHO initiated the "Quality Rights Initiative" in 2019 to reduce and eliminate coercive practices in mental health care. The training modules educate on human rights, mental health, legal capacity, recovery, and the right to freedom from coercion, violence, and abuse. The closing of state psychiatric hospitals has also led to "transinstitutionalization."

Transinstitutionalization

Transinstitutionalization is defined as the moving of psychiatric patients from one institution to another institution, such as nursing homes, prisons, community shelters, and forensic hospitals. If communities are unable to meet the needs of individuals who experience mental illness when discharged from psychiatric units in general hospitals, other avenues may be incorporated. Also, when U.S. state psychiatric hospitals close, many of their patients are placed in nursing homes. Thus, it could be viewed that we are just shifting costs for the care of individuals experiencing mental conditions from one entity to another by using both jails and nursing homes to house psychiatric clients.

Incarceration: Utilization of Penal Systems

There is a growing body of evidence that demonstrates the reinstitutionalization of clients with a mental illness by and through the states' penal systems; incarceration is being used for psychiatric-diagnosed individuals who are deemed unmanageable or noncompliant. Several areas of study have identified factors that contribute to incarceration. One is that, because of a mental illness, individuals may commit more criminal acts, thus facilitating potential incarceration. Research suggests that individuals experiencing a mental illness may be more prone to violence if they are actively experiencing delusions or have long-standing paranoia.[28] Other comorbidities include conditions such as substance misuse, homelessness, unemployment, and secondary effects of mental illness, such as cognitive impairment, that can compound the risk of committing a violent crime.[29] And two, individuals with a mental condition may intentionally commit lower-level crimes in order to sustain shelter. To stress again, the majority of researchers on this topic believe that those experiencing mental illness are more prone to being victims of crime versus being perpetrators.

United States

Statistics tabulated by the U.S. Department of Justice in 2012 revealed state prisoners with a mental condition were only slightly more likely to be serving time for a violent crime (50.6% for all mentally ill compared to 47.1% for inmates without a psychiatric diagnosis).[30] Individuals with an SMI were more likely (by 6%) to be in prison for a property crime and less likely for a drug offense.[31] It was also revealed during this particular study that homelessness was a frequent factor in the inmates' lives.

SAMHSA reported in 2023 that only 3% to 5% of violent acts can be attributed to individuals with an SMI.[32] Homicides over a 20-year period in the United States encompassed 388,311 individuals; an SMI diagnosis was attributed to 38,000 of those deaths.[33]

In 2018, the Bureau of Justice Statistics reported that 14% of prisoners in state and federal facilities met the criteria for having serious mental health conditions. In local jails, the number was 26%.[34] It is estimated that approximately two million people with mental illness are booked into prisons each year. According to the Prison Policy Initiative, in 2023, the percentage of people in state prisons who have been diagnosed with a mental disorder is 43%, and local jails are at 44%.[35] In Michigan, where mental illness afflicts a quarter of the state's 41,000 prisoners, it costs $95,000 a year to house each one, compared to $35,000 for prisoners without mental health problems.[36] The percentage of mental illness in U.S. prisons is exhibited in Figure 2.2.

Other Countries

The Australian Institute of Health and Welfare reported that in 2018, 40% of Australian prisoners identified as having previously been diagnosed with a mental

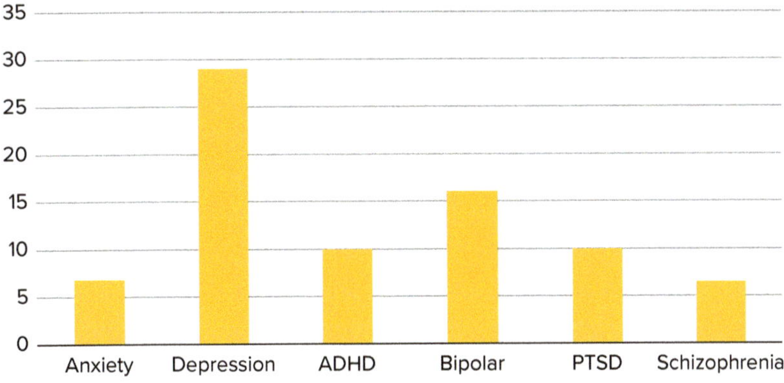

FIGURE 2.2 Percentage of Mental Illness in U.S. Prisons[37]

illness.[38] It was also identified that the prison environment can exacerbate mental illness symptoms and, in some cases, generate an inability for individuals to maintain their mental health. In the United Kingdom, the Mental Health Foundation estimates that up to 90% of British prisoners have a mental condition, substance misuse, or both.[39] In Canada, a schizophrenia diagnosis was attributed to 1.5% of inmates in general prisons and 2.2% in federal prisons.[40] A current study in French prisons revealed that there was a very high level of psychiatric conditions and substance misuse: substance misuse at 53.5%, suicide risk at 31.4%, anxiety disorder at 44.4%, psychotic syndromes at 6.9%, and major depressive disorder at 27.2%.[41] A global 2020 study of mental conditions regarding inmates is depicted in Figure 2.3.

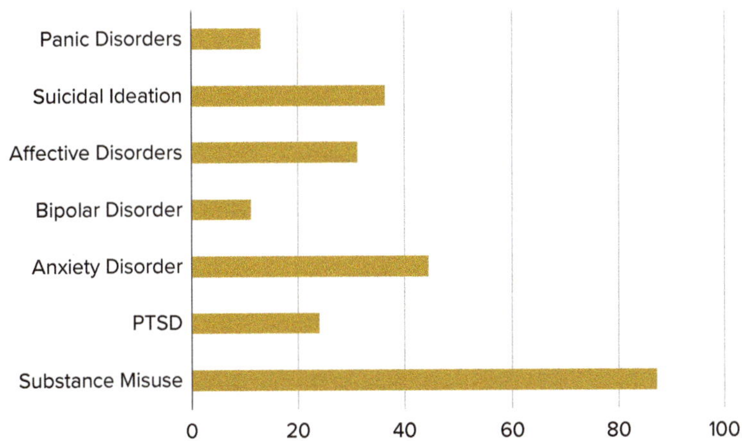

FIGURE 2.3 2020 Global Percentage of Inmates With Mental Conditions Incarcerated[42]

Mental Health Treatment While Incarcerated

Problems arise when adequate mental health services are not available in prisons. One study indicated that few jails provide a range of services, with most providing only intake screening and mental health evaluations (60% to 83% of the 10 jails surveyed).[43] It is estimated that approximately 63% of inmates do not receive mental health treatment while incarcerated in state and federal prisons,[44] and 50% of individuals do not receive their psychotropic medications while in prison.[45] The National Commission on Correctional Health Care identifies incarcerated basic health care services as group, psychosocial, psychoeducational, and individual counseling; crisis intervention; medication management; identification and referral; and treatment documentation and follow-up.[46]

Recidivism

There is ongoing research on the process of reducing recidivism. The mentally ill have been found to be 15% more likely to recidivate within 5 years.[47] Some communities have launched programs involving CMHCs and increased local law enforcement training to develop alternate interventions versus incarceration for minor criminal acts for individuals experiencing mental illness. For example, the state of Oregon has initiated the "Justice Reinvestment Initiative," which focuses on stopping the cycle of recidivism encompassing individuals with behavioral health needs and using treatment processes within community settings.[48]

The Forensic Assertive Community Treatment (FACT) service delivery model is for individuals with an SMI who are involved in the criminal justice system and builds on the evidence-based assertive community treatment model. FACT is designed to improve a client's mental health outcomes and daily functioning, reduce recidivism, divert individuals in need of mental health treatment away from the criminal justice system, manage costs, and increase public safety.[49]

Another study conducted in 2019 examined the correlation between accessibility to community-based mental health services and crime rates. The data suggests that increases in office-based mental health providers can reduce crime rates by 0.5%.[50] The National Bureau of Economic Research found that an increase of mental healthcare offices by 10 additional offices in a county reduces crime by 1.7% per 10,000 residents.[51]

Nursing Homes

Working around the Institute of Mental Disease rule is the reason why most states shifted the care of elderly diagnosed psychiatric clients in the United States to nursing homes located in community settings. On any given day, there are more than 500,000 people with a mental illness (excluding dementia) residing in U.S. nursing homes, greatly exceeding the number of all other healthcare institutions combined.[52] It could be viewed that nursing homes were and are another route of reinstitutionalization for individuals experiencing mental illness, thus establishing another venue of cost-shifting.

During the years 1969 to 1974, 1,263 patients were transferred from Bay State Hospital in Massachusetts to nursing homes.[53] From 1960 to 1980, in the United States, there was over a 100% increase in psychiatric conditions in nursing home populations.[54] It was estimated in 1994 that between 65% to 91% of nursing home residents had a significant mental disorder.[55] And that 19% of the residents admitted to nursing homes in 2005 were admitted with a mental condition other than dementia.[56] According to a recent study from the American Geriatrics Society, between 85% to 90% of nursing home residents have a mental or behavioral health problem.[57]

Other Countries

Psychiatric nursing homes were used in Norway from the 1950s to 2003; at the time of peak utilization, the average length of stay was 5 to 6 years.[58] It is estimated that 40% of Canadian nursing home residents had a mental disorder in 2021.[59] In 2018, it was suggested that 40% of residents living in care homes in the United Kingdom had significant depressive symptoms.[60] In a review of the records of 430,862 aged care residents 65 or older living in Australia, nearly 60% were found to have significant mental health difficulties, such as depressive, anxiety, or psychotic disorders, with the most common being depressive symptoms.[61] It is widely suggested that many other countries, besides the United States, transinstitutionalized patients into nursing homes with the closing of state-funded mental institutions.

Mental Health Treatment in Nursing Homes

A 2019 study of behavioral health services in U.S. nursing homes revealed that inadequate services were provided in one third of the facilities, with the major factor being a lack of staff education.[62] Of the 1,079 nursing homes in the study, there were employee concerns about admitting residents with behavioral health needs, including the need to devote more time to the residents, a concern for resident and staff safety, and perceived difficulties with sending residents back to the psychiatric hospitals.[63]

In some regions in the United States, there is also a shortage of behavioral health specialists to make rounds in nursing homes to establish adequate assessment and treatment processes. Many nursing homes have contracted with psychiatric mental health nurse practitioners associated with behavioral service units in general hospitals to meet their residents' mental health care needs. These nurses make rounds in nursing homes once a month to assess residents and provide recommendations for current and ongoing treatment. Setting up this type of system in nursing homes develops collaboration with the community behavioral health unit, improving resident quality of care. In communities that lack behavioral nurse practitioners and/or adequate numbers of psychiatrists/psychologists, primary care providers and the social service department can address residents' mental health needs.

Nursing Home Closures

Another dilemma in this situation is the closing of nursing homes in the United States, as portrayed in Figure 2.4. From 2015 to 2019, 4% of the nursing homes in the United States closed approximately 550 facilities.[64] The development of assisted living facilities and increased home health options have reduced the number of individuals who require long-term care and/or skilled care services. There is a developing trend in thinking to deinstitutionalize nursing homes.

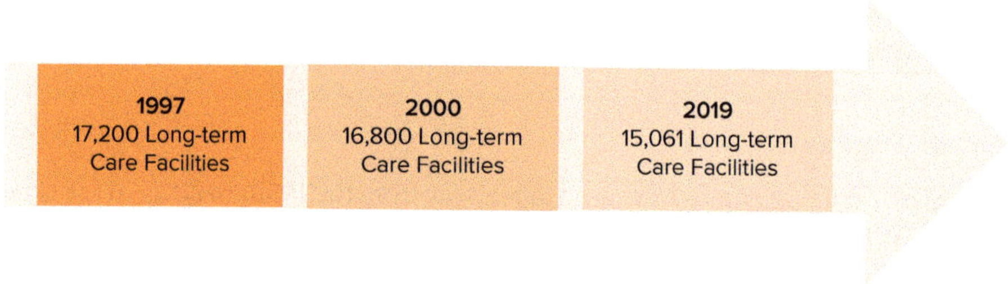

1997	2000	2019
17,200 Long-term Care Facilities	16,800 Long-term Care Facilities	15,061 Long-term Care Facilities

FIGURE 2.4 Closing of Nursing Homes in America

The COVID-19 pandemic generated additional operating strains on nursing homes, with 143 closures and mergers occurring in 2020, and a projected change in nursing home operations was forecasted for 1,670 facilities in 2021.[65] A survey conducted by the American Healthcare Association and National Center for Assisted Living revealed that approximately 66% of nursing homes said they could close in 2021 due to operating at a revenue loss.[66] It is estimated that between 300 to 400 additional nursing homes closed in the United States between 2021 and 2022 and that nursing homes in many other countries faced similar situations.

Forensic Hospitals

Forensic hospitals are described as secure healthcare institutions that are used for individuals who have a criminal record and/or SMI that are at risk for serious violence. Forensic mental health services of assessment and treatment are provided to these individuals when recommended by courts, law enforcement, justice agencies, or other mental health services.

Assessment processes may entail whether the person is capable of making a plea in court, the state of mind of the patient at the time of a crime, and the current need for psychiatric treatment. These hospitals offer long stay periods, typically 2 to 3 years, for individuals who are perceived as unsafe to live in society. It has been suggested by many researchers examining the global mental healthcare crisis that these institutions are being used as a transinstitutional process.

A study in Austria concluded that an increase in admission rates to forensic hospitals was related to inadequate provision of comprehensive care for "difficult" but not extremely dangerous psychotic patients living in the community.[67] This development, which can be observed in nearly all European countries, raises concerns with regard to efforts to destigmatize both patients and psychiatry.[68] It has been argued that this trend in Western Europe and the United States is also partially attributed to the continual decline of general psychiatric beds available. A 2020 analysis revealed that, while the number of forensic beds and the duration of forensic psychiatric treatment have increased in several European Union states, this is not observed in others. Patient demographics, average lengths of stay and legal frameworks also differ substantially.[69]

According to the National Institute of Mental Health, in 2021, one in five adults or 57.8 million individuals, experienced a mental illness.[70] In 2019, the Centers for Disease Control and Prevention (CDC) reported that the percentage of noninstitutionalized adults who experienced serious psychological distress (regular feelings of nervousness, anxiety, and worry) within 30 days of the survey was 11.2%.[71] Medical visits in 2018 related to individuals diagnosed with mental conditions encompassed 55.7 million individuals in the United States.[72] The number of emergency department visits with mental disorders, behavioral, and neurodevelopmental as the primary diagnosis was 6.2 million in 2020.[73] This large population impacted by mental health adversities substantiates the necessity for adequate and improved community-based mental health treatment systems.

There are many factors that have evolved with the closing of state psychiatric institutions that have established cracks in the mental healthcare system for clients to fall through and not receive the services they so desperately need. Hopefully, in time, we can fill those cracks and provide mental health services globally that facilitate recovery, eradicate retraumatization, and maintain well-being in a community-based setting for those experiencing mental conditions. In the subsequent chapters, we will examine the mental healthcare crisis and how we can bridge the gap between community-based services and brief general hospital psychiatric unit stays.

BOX 2.1 A Critical Thinking Synopsis—Do You Agree?

The process of deinstitutionalization of the mentally ill has been occurring globally for decades. We have examined the perceived beneficial aspects of this worldwide change in perceptions of required services for mental health decline, which many people believe establishes a more "humane" and cost-effective delivery of mental health care. But, as discussed, transinstitutionalization and the lack of establishment of adequate community-based mental health services have evolved into some negative impacts for mental health care recipients, which will be explained in more depth in later chapters.

Based on the author's experience of being employed in a psychiatric institution for 10 years, deinstitutionalization is a healthier process for those clients who can be managed in a community setting, assisting in recovering from mental health decline more efficiently without the added burdens of institutional environments. Now, in instances of violence (suicidal, homicidal,

(*continued*)

self-harming behaviors), crisis intervention, which includes institutionalization or admission to a behavioral crisis unit to sustain safety, may need to be incorporated. And those individuals who are unable to be managed and are deemed to be unsafe may require lifetime institutionalization to maintain societal well-being.

Main Points

1. Deinstitutionalization, which began in 1955, is explained as the discharging of patients from psychiatric hospitals and the subsequent partial or full closure of the institutions. It has been identified that there are essentially three major reasons for this global process occurring: money, new psychotropic medications available, and poorly perceived reputations of the institutions.
2. There have been many established positive aspects identified with the closing of state-funded psychiatric facilities: better quality of life through improved living conditions, an improvement in life skills, promotion of human and civil rights, increased family involvement, improved focus on treatment, social inclusion, and a decreased potential for revictimization.
3. The closing of psychiatric hospitals has also led to "transinstitutionalization." Transinstitutionalization is defined as the moving of psychiatric patients from one institution to another institution, such as nursing homes, prisons, community shelters, and forensic hospitals.

Notes

1. Tabler, Dave (2008), 125 Reasons you'll get sent to the Lunatic Asylum, Appalachian History, https://apalachianhistory.net/2008/12/125-reasons-youll-get-sent-to-lunatic-html (accessed July 10, 2019).
2. Estren, Mark (2013), *Prescription drug abuse,* Ronin Publishing, Inc., pp. 28.
3. Eide, Stephen (2018), Systems under strain: Deinstitutionalization in New York State and City, Manhattan Institute, https://www.manhattan-institute.org/deinstitutionalization-mental-illness-new-york-state-city. (accessed November 12, 2021).
4. Placzek, Jessica (2016), Did the emptying of mental hospitals contribute to homelessness? https://www.kqed.org/news/11209729/did-the-emptying-of-mental-hospitaks-contribute-to-homelessness (accessed November 12, 2021).
5. Hospital Review (2016), Amid shortage, number of psychiatric beds down 10 percent from 2010, https://www.beckerhospitalreview.com/amid-shortage-number-of-psychiatric-beds-down-10-percent (accessed April 30, 2021).
6. Michas, Frederic (2022), Mental health treatment facilities by setting services in the U.S. 2020, Statista, https://www.statista.com/statistics/450877/mental-health-facilities-in-the-us-by-service-type (accessed April 24, 2022).

7. National Alliance on Mental Illness (2021), Mental health by the numbers, https://nami.org/mhstats (accessed October 22, 2021).

8. Mental Health America (2022), Access to care data/ranking, https://mhanational.org/issues/2022/mental-health-america-access-care-data (accessed August 18, 2023).

9. Mundt, Adrian, et al. (2022), *Minimum and optimal numbers of psychiatric beds: Expert consensus using Delphi process, Molecular Psychiatry,* 27, https://doi.org/10.1038/s41380-021-01435-0 (accessed August 18, 2023), pp. 1873–1879.

10. Mundt, Adrian, et al. (2022), *Minimum and optimal numbers of psychiatric beds: Expert consensus using Delphi process, Molecular Psychiatry,* 27, https://doi.org/10.1038/s41380-021-01435-0 (accessed August 18, 2023), pp. 1873–1879.

11. Wikipedia (2022), Category: Psychiatric hospitals by country, https://www.en.wikipedia.org/wiki/category:psychiatric_hospitals_by_country (accessed April 30, 2022).

12. Eurostat Statistics Explained (2018), Hospital beds by type of care, https://www.ec.europa.eu/eurostat/statistics-explained/index.php?title=healthcare_resource_statistics_beds (accessed November 13, 2021).

13. Eurostat Statistics Explained (2018), Hospital beds by type of care, https://www.ec.europa.eu/eurostat/statistics-explained/index.php?title=healthcare_resource_statistics_beds (accessed November 13, 2021).

14. Eurostat Statistics Explained (2018), Hospital beds by type of care, https://www.ec.europa.eu/eurostat/statistics-explained/index.php?title=healthcare_resource_statistics_beds (accessed November 13, 2021).

15. Scaly, Patricia, PhD, and Whitehead, Paul, PhD (2004), *Forty years of deinstitutionalization of psychiatric services in Canada: An Empirical Assessment, Can J Psychiatry,* Vol. 49, No. 4. https://pubmed.ncbi.nlm.nih.gov/15147023/ (accessed November 13, 2021). pp. 250.

16. Moroz, Nicholas, MPH (2020), *Mental health services in Canada: Barriers and cost-effective solutions to increase access,* https://doi.org/10.1177/0840470420933911 (accessed November 13, 2021).

17. Olsen, Deidre (2022), We explain how to access different mental health services in Germany, as well as private health insurance, emergency support, and more, https://www.expatica.com/de/healthcare-services/mental-health-in-germany-346138 (accessed September 4, 2022).

18. Rossa-Roccor, Verna, et al. (2020), Victimization of people with severe mental illness outside and within the mental health care system: Results on prevalence and risk factors from a multicenter study, *Front Psychiatry,* 11:563860, https://doi.org/10.3389/fpsyt.2020.563860 (accessed November 14, 2021).

19. Sinclair, Elizabeth (2018), Research weekly: Violence in hospitals by people with serious mental illness, Treatment Advocacy Center, https://advocacycenter.org/fixing-the-system/features-and-news (accessed November 14, 2021).

20. Ulrich, Roger and Lundin, Stefan (2018), Psychiatric ward design can reduce aggressive Behavior, *Journal of Environmental Psychology,* 57, https://doi.org/10.1016/j/jenvp/2018/05/002 (accessed November 14, 2021), pp. 53–66.

21. Weltens, Irene, et al. (2021), Aggression on the psychiatric ward: Prevalence and risk factors. A systematic review of the literature, *PLoS One,* 18(10):e0258346, https:/doi.org/10.1371/journal.pone.0268346, https://pubmed.ncbi.nlm.nih.gov/34624057 (accessed December 5, 2021).

22. Barnett, Brian, MD (2020), *Addressing sexual violence in psychiatric facilities*, Psychiatry Online, https://doi.org/10.1176/appi.ps.202000038 (accessed November 14, 2021).
23. Barnett, Brian, MD (2020), *Addressing sexual violence in psychiatric facilities*, Psychiatry Online, https://doi.org/10.1176/appi.ps.202000038 (accessed November 14, 2021).
24. Barnett, Brian, MD (2020), *Addressing sexual violence in psychiatric facilities*, Psychiatry Online, https://doi.org/10.1176/appi.ps.202000038 (accessed November 14, 2021).
25. Kersting, Xenia, et al. (2019), Physical harm and death in the context of coercive measures in psychiatric patients: A systematic review, *Frontiers in Psychiatry*, https://doi.org/10.3389/fpsyt.2019.00400 (accessed November 14, 2021).
26. Kersting, Xenia, et al. (2019), Physical harm and death in the context of coercive measures in psychiatric patients: A systematic review, *Frontiers in Psychiatry*, https://doi.org/10.3389/fpsyt.2019.00400 (accessed November 14, 2021).
27. Kersting, Xenia, et al. (2019), Physical harm and death in the context of coercive measures in psychiatric patients: A systematic review, *Frontiers in Psychiatry*, https://doi.org/10.3389/fpsyt.2019.00400 (accessed November 14, 2021).
28. Ghiasi, Norman., et al. (2021), Psychiatric illness and criminality, StatPearls, https://pubmed.ncbi.nlm. nih.gov/30726749/ (accessed November 21, 2021).
29. Ghiasi, Norman., et al. (2021), Psychiatric illness and criminality, StatPearls, https://pubmed.ncbi.nlm.nih.gov/30726749/ (accessed November 21, 2021).
30. Raphael, Steven and Stoll, Michael (2014), Assessing the contribution of the deinstitutionalization of the mentally ill to growth in the U.S. incarceration rate, *The Journal of Legal Studies*, 42(1), https://ideas.repec.org/a/ucp/jlstud/doi10.1086-667773.html#:~:text=Our%20estimates%20suggest%20that%204-7%20percent%20of%20incarceration,would%20not%20have%20been%20incarcerated%20in%20years%20past (accessed November 21, 2021), pp. 187–222.
31. Raphael, Steven and Stoll, Michael (2014), Assessing the contribution of the deinstitutionalization of the mentally ill to Growth in the U.S. incarceration rate, *The Journal of Legal Studies*, 42(1), https://ideas.repec.org/a/ucp/jlstud/doi10.1086-667773.html#:~:text=Our%20estimates%20suggest%20that%204-7%20percent%20of%20incarceration,would%20not%20have%20been%20incarcerated%20in%20years%20past (accessed November 21, 2021), pp. 187–222.
32. SAMHSA (2023), Mental health myths and facts, https://www.samhsa.gov/mental-health/myths-and-facts (accessed August 18, 2023).
33. Mental illness Policy (2012), New study suggests that severely mentally ill individuals who are not being treated are responsible for 10 percent of U.S. homicides, https://www.mentalillnesspolicy.org/consequences/1000-homicides.html (accessed November 21, 2021).
34. Lyon, Ed (2019), *Imprisoning America's mentally ill*, Prison Legal News, https://www.prisonlegalnews.org/news/2019/feb/4/imprisoning-americas-mentally-ill/ (accessed November 15, 2021).
35. Prison Policy Initiative (2023), Mental health: Policies and practices surrounding mental health, https://www.prisonpolicy.org/research/mental_health/ (accessed August 18, 2023).
36. Lyon, Ed (2019), *Imprisoning America's mentally ill*, Prison Legal News, https://www.prisonlegalnews.org/news/2019/feb/4/imprisoning-americas-mentally-ill/ (accessed November 15, 2021).

37. Prins, Seth, MPH (2014), *Prevalence of mental illness in U.S. State prisons: A systematic review,* https://doi.org/10.1176/appi.ps.20130066 (accessed April 30, 2022).

38. Gallant Law (2019), Mental illness and crime: What's the link? https://www.gallantlaw.com.au/mental-llness-and-crime-whats-the-link/ (accessed November 21, 2021).

39. Schwarzwalder, Alejandro (2017), Mental disorder and crime, https://wwwantoniocasella.eu/archipsy/schwarzwalder_2017.pdf (accessed November 21, 2021).

40. Schwarzwalder, Alejandro (2017), Mental disorder and crime, https://wwwantoniocasella.eu/archipsy/schwarzwalder_2017.pdf, (accessed November 21, 2021).

41. Fovet, Thomas, et al. (2020), Mental disorders on admission to jail: A study of prevalence and a comparison with community sample in the north of France, *Forensic Science International: Mind and Law,* https://journals.elsevier.com/forensic-science-international-mind-and-law (accessed November 21, 2021).

42. Gomez-Figueroa, Helen, and Camino-Proano, Armando (2022), *Mental and behavioral disorders in prison context, rev esp Sanid Penit,* 24 (2), https://www.ncbi.nlm.nih.gov/pmc/articles/PMC9578298 (accessed August 18, 2023), pp. 66–74.

43. Agency for Healthcare Research and Quality (2012), Interventions for adults with serious mental illness who are involved in the criminal justice system, https://www.healthcare.ahrq.gov/products/mental-illness-adults-prisons/research-protocol. (accessed November 15, 2021).

44. National Alliance on Mental Illness (2023), Mental health treatment while incarcerated, https://www.nami.org/advocacy/policy-priorities/improving-health/mental-health-treatment-while-incarcerated (accessed August 15, 2023).

45. National Alliance on Mental Illness (2023), Mental health treatment while incarcerated, https://www.nami.org/advocacy/policy-priorities/improving-health/mental-health-treatment-while-incarcerated (accessed August 15, 2023).

46. National Commission on Correctional Healthcare (2021), Basic mental health services, https://www.ncchc.org/spotlight-on-the-standards/basic-mental-health-services (accessed November 15, 2021).

47. Bliss, Kevin (2020), *Mental health and prison systems in major need of reform,* Prison Legal News, https://www.prisonlegalnews.org/news/2020/oct/1/mental-health-and-prison-systems-major-need-reform/ (accessed November 15, 2021).

48. Cowie, Robb (2018), *Oregon kicks off data-driven review of state's criminal justice, behavioral health systems,* https://www.oregon.gov/oha/ERD/pages/oregon-kicks-off-data-driven-review-of-states-crminal-justice-behavioral-health-systems (accessed November 15, 2021).

49. SAMHSA (2018), Forensic assertive community treatment action brief, https://store.samhsa.gov/sites/default/files/d7/priv/pe p19-fact-br.pdf (accessed August 18, 2023), pp.1–8.

50. Deza, Monica, et al. (2020), *Local access to mental healthcare and crime,* https://www.nber.org/papers/w27619 (accessed November 21, 2021).

51. Deza, Monica, et al. (2020), *Local access to mental healthcare and crime,* https://www.nber.org/papers/w27619 (accessed November 21, 2021).

52. Aschbrenner, Kelly PhD, et al. (2011), Nursing homes admissions and long-stay conversions among persons with and without serious mental illness, *Journal of Aging and Social Policy,* https:/doi.org/10.1080/08959420/2011/579511, https://pubmed.ncbi.nlm.nih.gov/21740203/ (accessed November 15, 2021), pp. 286–304.

53. Phillips, Andrew, (1978), The *role of nursing homes in the deinstitutionalization of psychiatric patients from state hospitals,* https://www.scholarworks.umass.edudissertation_1/3431/# (accessed November 16, 2021).

54. Loewenstein, Nina, JD, MPH (2019), *The inappropriate institutionalization of people with mental illness in long-term care,* https://www.nuraunghome411.org/wp-content/uploads/2021/02/webinar.institutionalization.02162021.pdf (accessed November 19, 2021).

55. Grabowski, David, MA, et al. (2010), Quality of mental health care for nursing home residents: A literature review, *Med Care Res Rev,* 67(6): doi.10.1177/1077558710362538, https://pubmed.ncbi.nlm.nih.gov/20223943. (accessed November 16, 2021), pp. 627–656.

56. Grabowski, David, MA, et al. (2010), Quality of mental health care for nursing home residents: A literature review, *Med Care Res Rev,* 67(6): doi.10.1177/1077558710362538, https://pubmed.ncbi.nlm.nih.gov/20223943 (accessed November 16, 2021), pp. 627–656.

57. Nursing Home Abuse Justice (2022), Mental health in nursing homes: Managing emotional health, https://www.nursinghomeabuse.org/resources/nursing-home-mental-health (accessed April 24, 2022).

58. Pedersen, Bernhard and Kolstad, Arnulf (2009), De-institutionalization and trans-institutionalization-changing trends of inpatient care in Norwegian mental health institutions 1950–2007, *International Journal of Mental Health Systems,* 3(28). https://doi.org/10.1186/1752-4458-3-28, https://pubmed.ncbi.nlm.nih.gov/200356231/ (accessed November 16, 2021).

59. Kehyayan, Vahe, et al. (2021), Profile of residents with mental disorders in Canadian long-term care facilities: A cross–sectional study, *Journal of Long-Term Care,* https://journal.ilpnetwork.org/articles/10.31389/jltc.47, pp. 154–156.

60. Potter, Rachel, PhD, et al. (2018), The impact of the physical environment on depressive symptoms of older residents living in care homes: A mixed methods study, *The Gerontologist,* 58(3), https://doi.org/10.1093/geront/gnx041 (accessed August 18, 2023), pp. 438–447.

61. Bhar, Sunil, et al. (2022), Addressing mental health in aged care residents, *Advances in Psychiatry and Mental Health,* 2(1), https://doi.org/10.1016/j.ypsc.2022.06.002, pp. 183–191.

62. Orth, Jessica, MS, MPH, et al. (2019), Providing behavioral health services in nursing homes is difficult: Findings from a national survey, *Journal of American Geriatrics Society,* 67(8), https://pubmed.ncbi.nlm.nih.gov/31166614. (accessed April 25, 2022), pp. 1713–1717.

63. Spanko, Alex (2019), *Even as demands rises, nursing homes face major behavioral health hurdles,* https://www.skillednursingnews.com/2019/06/depite-demands-nursing-homes-face-major-behavioral-health-hurdles (accessed November 16, 2021).

64. Gleckman, Howard (2020), *Why are so many nursing homes shutting down?* https://www.forbes.com/sites/howardgleckman/2020/93/02/why-are-so-many-nursing-homes-shutting-down/?sh=6d (accessed November 16, 2021).

65. Kelley, Alexandra (2021), *About 25 percent of nursing homes to survive in 2021,* https://www.thehill.com/changing-america/well-being/longevity/560820 (accessed November 16, 2021).

66. American Health Law Associate (2020), *Two thirds of nursing homes say they may close in 2021 due to COVID-19 costs, survey demonstrates,* https://www.americanhealthlaw.org/content-library/ahla/daily/article/5b4b8c16-ca93-4f84-9e2a-d9bfb396e15c/ (accessed November 16, 2021).

67. Schanda, Hans, et al. (2009), Dangerous or merely difficult? The new population of forensic mental hospitals, *European Psychiatry,* 24(6), https://doi.org/10.1016/j.eurpsy.2009.07.006, https://pubmed.ncbi.nlm.nih.gov/19717282/ (accessed April 24, 2022), pp. 365–372.

68. Schanda, Hans, et al. (2009), Dangerous or merely difficult? The new population of forensic mental hospitals, *European Psychiatry,* 24(6), https://doi.org/10.1016/j.eurpsy.2009.07.006, https://pubmed.ncbi.nlm.nih.gov/19717282/ (accessed April 24, 2022), pp. 365–372.

69. Tomlin, Jack, et al. (2021), Forensic mental health in Europe: Some key figures, *Social Psychiatry and Psychiatric Epidemiology,* 56(1), https://doi.org/10.1007/s00127-020-01909-6 (accessed April 24, 2022), pp. 108–117.

70. National Institute of Mental Health (2022), *Mental illness,* https://www.nimh.nih.gov/health/statistics/mental-illness (accessed August 18, 2023).

71. Clarke, Tainya, PhD, et al. (2020), *Early release of selected estimates based on data from the 2019 national health interview survey,* Division of Health Interview Statistics. National Center for Health Statistics. U.S. Department of Health and Human Services, Centers for Disease Control and Prevention, https://www.cdc.gov/nchs/data/nhis/earlyrelease/EarlyRelease202009-508.pdf (accessed April 22,2021), pp. 1–2.

72. Okeyode, Santo (2018), *National ambulatory medical care survey: 2018 national summary tables,* National Center for Health Statistics, U. S. Department of Health and Human Services. Centers for Disease Control and Prevention, https://www.cdc.gov/nchs/data/ahcd/namcs_summary/2018_namcs_web_tables.pdf (accessed April 22,2021), pp. 1–40.

73. Center for Disease Control and Prevention (2023), Mental Illness, https://www.cdc.gov/nchs/fastats/mental-health.htm (accessed August 18, 2023).

Credits

Fig. 2.1: Data Source: https://en.wikipedia.org/wiki/Category:Psychiatric_hospitals_by_country.

Fig. 2.2: Data Source: Seth J. Prins, "The Prevalence of Mental Illnesses in U.S. State Prisons: A Systematic Review," Psychiatric Services, vol. 65, no. 7, American Psychiatric Association Publishing, 2014.

PART II

IMPACTS, DISCREPANCIES, AND ADVERSITIES

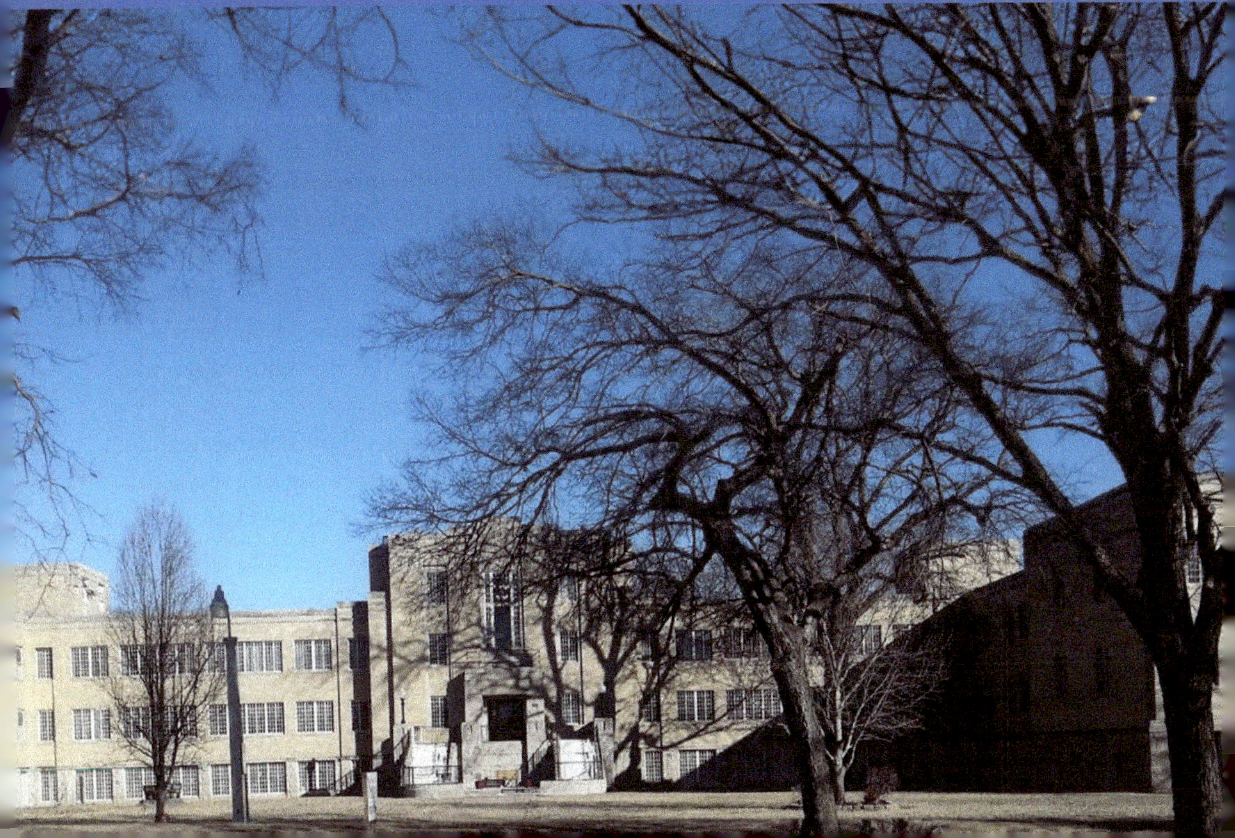

CHAPTER 3

Mental Health Professionals

The main objective of this chapter is for the reader to obtain greater clarity on mental health care workforce shortages and their impact on the delivery of mental health services.

Mental health professionals encompass psychiatrists, psychologists, nurses, technicians, counselors, nurse practitioners, therapists, etc. Individuals employed in the mental health field can assist clients in understanding and coping with thoughts, feelings, and behaviors, offer guidance, and assess/diagnose/treat mental health conditions. The goal of mental health treatment is to improve a patient's mental health. Global mental health workforce shortages are profound in many countries; in this chapter, we will examine statistics on health care worker shortages, perceived reasons for the dilemma, and how the shortages can impact mental health care recipients. Additionally, we will expound on the therapeutic relationship, evidence-based care, and legalities related to this branch of medicine.

Psychiatrists and Psychologists

Psychiatrists and psychologists have existed globally for centuries; Wilhelm Wundt (1832–1920) was considered the first psychologist,[1] and Johann Weyer (1515–1588) was the first physician to specialize in mental illness.[2] Psychiatrists and psychologists have similar practices, yet they are different. Psychiatrists are medical doctors who can prescribe medications, diagnose illnesses, manage treatment regimens, and provide therapies for mental illnesses. Psychologists primarily provide psychotherapy and behavioral guidance to clients; they are not medical doctors.

Worldwide, there has been a steady decline in individuals choosing the mental health branch of medicine as a career choice. Currently, there is ongoing research being conducted regarding the number of psychiatrists and psychologists decreasing globally.

Mental Health Practitioner Shortages

WHO reported in 2015 that nearly half of the world's population lives in a country where there is less than one psychiatrist per 100,000 people.[3] Statista reiterated this number in 2020 (1.7 psychiatrists) and further elaborated that there are 1.4 psychologists per 100,000 people globally.[4] Figure 3.1 depicts the number of psychiatrists in several countries.

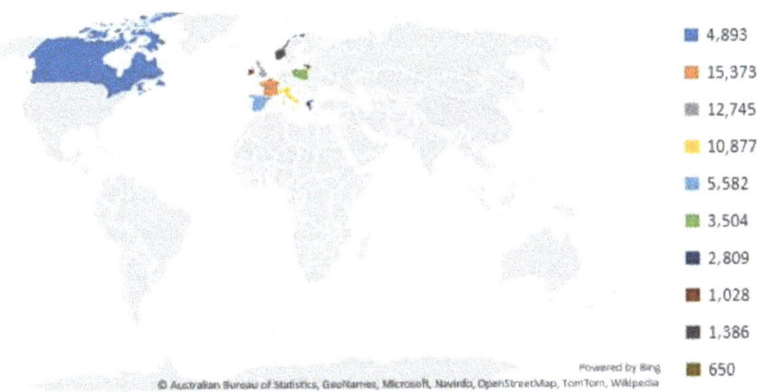

FIGURE 3.1 Number of Psychiatrists[5, 6]

United States

In the United States, it is estimated that, in 2021, over one third of Americans lived in an area lacking mental health care practitioners.[7] In some states, over 80% of the population lives in a mental health professional shortage area.[8] One earlier study estimated the shortage encompassed 6,471 psychiatrists, affecting approximately 124 million people.[9] Another 2018 report by Merritt Hawkins revealed that there were 30,451 practicing psychiatrists in the United States, which is about nine psychiatrists per 100,000 Americans.[10] The most recent data in the United States indicates there are 26,500 practicing psychiatrists in the country, with a current population of 339.9 million.[11]

There is also a continuous decline in practicing psychologists in the United States; currently, there are approximately 63,579 licensed psychologists,[12] with approximately 33% of the counties having no records of a licensed psychologist. The Bureau of Labor estimated in 2022, that there were approximately 14,100 psychologist positions that open each year in America.[13]

The shortage of both psychiatrists and psychologists appears to be more pronounced in rural regions in the United States versus urban populations. It is believed that the Affordable Care Act in the United States increased the number of individuals who can now obtain mental health care services, and potentially, this process has also contributed to the ongoing shortage of availability of practicing psychiatrists to treat patients, especially in rural regions, because of increased caseloads. Anna Ratzcliff, MD, PhD, psychiatry residency program director at the University of Washington in Seattle, stated that several factors fuel the shortage: "The U.S. population has grown, there's a lot of mental health need, especially with the pandemic, and we don't have enough residency slots to train people."[14]

The U.S. Government Accountability Office released a report to Congress in October of 2022 titled *Behavioral Health, Available Workforce Information and Federal Actions to Help Recruit and Retain Providers*; the office identified three barriers to the crisis: financial, educational, and workplace. The goals for the position paper are financial assistance for education, early outreach and mentorship, and leveraging the existing workforce through telehealth.[15]

In 2021, there was an increase in the number (1,537 students) of allopathic and osteopathic seniors choosing to enter psychiatry, compared to 685 students in 2014.[16] Art Walaszek, MD, a psychiatrist at the University of Wisconsin School of Medicine and Public Health in Madison, stated, "Creating new residency slots is critical. After all, it's the only way to produce more psychiatrists."[17]

Other Countries

A psychiatry shortage is pervasive in Ontario and more widely across Canada, and it is believed this will continue.[18] It is estimated that the number of psychiatrists per population is expected to decrease by 15% by 2030.[19] The United Kingdom is also exhibiting mental health professional shortages. England has just one consultant psychiatrist for every 12,600 people, and services are unable to meet the recorded demand for treatment, according to the Royal College of Psychiatrists.[20] There is also a critical shortage of psychiatrists in Australia, which was to some extent acknowledged in the 2021 federal budget through the investment of $11 million into 30 new psychiatry training programs by 2023.[21]

Another reason for the shortage of both psychiatrists and psychologists globally can be attributed to an aging workforce and fewer individuals pursuing mental health as a career choice because of lower rates of reimbursement, increased documentation obligations, and regulatory requirements. Globally, fewer and fewer medical students have been going into mental health for their field of practice.

The ongoing dilemma of mental health practitioner shortages contributes to the mental healthcare crisis being experienced globally due to the lack of availability of adequate numbers of psychiatrists/psychologists to treat clients. Saul Levin, MD, CEO, and medical director of the American Psychiatric Association, stated,

> People can't get care. It affects their lives, their ability to work, to socialize, or even to get out of bed.[22]

Shortages of mental health care workers exist in other areas also, such as counselors, therapists, psychiatric technicians and nurses.

Counselors, Therapists, Technicians

Psychiatric technicians are individuals who work directly with mental health clients in psychiatric hospitals, residential mental health facilities and other mental health establishments who assist with daily activities, therapeutic care, and monitoring of patients under the supervision of psychiatrists, psychologists, and nurses. In Missouri, within the Department of Mental Health's Division in 2021, approximately 32% of entry-level psychiatric technician positions were vacant.[23] The Bureau of Labor projects that employment for psychiatric techs will grow 9% from 2021 to 2031.[24]

Licensed professional counselors are mental health service providers with a master's or doctorate degree who work with individuals treating mental, behavioral, and emotional conditions. An estimate in 2022, is that there were over 109,664 mental health counselors employed in the United States.[25] There were approximately 54,800 marriage and family therapists in the nation.[26] And, there were approximately 188,401 licensed social workers practicing in the United States.[27] Most counselors in the United States have stated that they are unable to accept new clients due to an already existing workload.

The population in the United States in 2023 was 339.9 million; according to the CDC, more than 50% of the U.S. population will be diagnosed with a mental illness or disorder at some point in their lifetime.[28] The numbers speak for themselves with regard to the extent of the problem; there are not enough mental health care workers to meet the needs of people. Figure 3.2 depicts mental health professional shortages in U.S. counties. In 2022, no state was without some shortage areas in their counties, and the problem has been prevalent for many years.

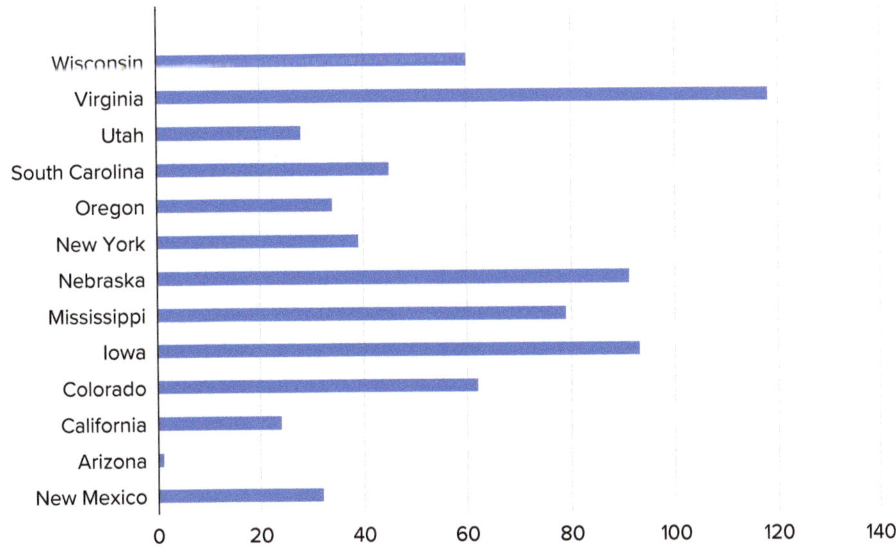

FIGURE 3.2 U.S. Mental Health Care Professional Shortages[29]

I found several articles that reported that there was a shortage of counselors, therapists, and psychiatric technicians throughout the European Union and other countries, but none that provided specifics on the actual percentage or number of behavioral health staff needed or actually employed. Worldwide, psychiatric nursing is practiced as a separate branch of nursing that was established centuries ago; next, we will examine the nurse's role in mental health care to illustrate how shortages of nurses can impact mental health care recipients.

Psychiatric Nursing

Mental health nursing is a branch of the nursing profession that entails caring for patients with mental illness and/or distress. Psychiatric nursing was recognized as a necessity for the establishment of quality patient care in the early 1900s. But the history of mental health nursing can be traced back to ancient philosophical thinkers; Marcos Tullius Cicero (a Roman philosopher, 106 BC–43 BC) was the first known person to create a questionnaire for clients experiencing mental illness, using biographical information to determine the best course of treatment and care.[30]

Psychiatrist Dr. William Ellis, in his 1836 publication *Treatise on Insanity*, openly stated that an established mental health nursing practice calmed depressed patients and gave hope to the hopeless.[31] Historically, psychiatric nursing practice has been influenced by traditional wisdom passed down through generations by word of mouth and in published textbooks.[32] Much of this nursing care has been based on personal experience, experiences of past nurses, and others who have gone before them.[33] It is believed by some that current mental health nursing practice is still grounded in tradition, unsystematic trial and error, and authority.[34]

Training

As stated earlier, in 1880, McLean Hospital became the first hospital-housed school for the training of psychiatric nurses in the United States. Boston City College (the first outside school to educate nurses in mental health care) was established by Linda Richards in 1882, and psychiatric nursing was officially formalized through this process.[35] Linda Richards is considered to be the first American psychiatric nurse.

Mental health nursing education was then established as part of the general nursing school curriculum at Johns Hopkins University in 1913. The first psychiatric nursing textbook, *Nursing Mental Diseases*, by Harriet Bailey, was published in 1920.[36] The National Mental Health Act recognized psychiatric nursing as one of the four core mental health disciplines in 1946. Rutgers University, in 1954, then established the first psychiatric nursing graduate program, leading to the foundation of the American Psychiatric Nurses Association in 1986.

In 1891, England established certification (in-service training) for psychiatric nurses by and through the Medico-Psychological Association.[37] Canada established its first regular mental health training programs for nurses in 1921 at the asylum in Brandon, Manitoba.[38] The Dutch Nursing Law of 1921 established a psychiatric diploma, route B process in their nurses training programs, offering more years of specialized training.[39]

Psychiatric Mental Health Nurse Practitioner (PMHNP)

PMHNPs are nurses trained to provide mental health services to individuals across the life span in various inpatient and outpatient settings. The role of the PMHNP can include providing therapy and prescribing medications, performing physical and psychosocial assessments, educating families and caregivers, establishing diagnoses, providing case management, and conducting emergency psychiatric care and treatment effectiveness evaluations. A master's in science in nursing is the minimum requirement for nurse practitioners; that typically takes two years (a bachelor's in science in nursing is a requirement to enter a program) to complete.

As discussed earlier in the transinstitutionalization section, many nursing homes use PMHNPs for their residents' mental health care, and these nurses routinely visit the post-acute care facilities, seeing both short-term and long-term clients. It is estimated that there are 10,474 PMHNPs in the United States.[40]

A study published in *Health Affairs* in 2022 found that in 2019, nearly one in three mental health prescriber visits to Medicare patients were done by psychiatric nurse practitioners.[41] Psychiatrists billing Medicare dropped by 6% between 2011 and 2019, but the number of psychiatric nurse practitioners increased by 162%.[42] PMHNPs are assisting in closing the gap between the demand for mental health services and access to care. PMHNPs are used in several other countries, including Australia, Canada, Sweden, the United Kingdom, and the Netherlands; these countries experience nurse shortages also.

Nurse Shortages

Nursing mental health delivery systems have been impacted on numerous levels for many years. One major issue is that the number of nurses entering the psychiatric branch of medicine has been decreasing globally. In 2021, there were approximately 41,290 behavioral/mental health nurses employed in the United States.[43] It has been relayed by some individuals who have studied the mental healthcare crisis that a general lack of interest in psychiatric nursing is the major contributing factor to the shortage. There is also the risk of personal injury and legal/ethical dilemmas in this branch of medicine that potentially impact nurses choosing psychiatric nursing as a career choice.

At present date, it is estimated that globally there are 3.8 mental health care nurses per 100,000 people.[44] Approximately 9.1 million people in Canada will be affected by a mental illness during their lifetime, while Canada has 6,000 registered psychiatric nurses currently employed.[45] In Spain, there are 2.87 mental health nurses per 100,000 people.[46] England had approximately 39,000 full-time mental health nurses employed in 2021,[47] while it is estimated that 30% (20 million) of the United Kingdom's population suffers from at least one mental condition. With approximately one billion people living with a mental condition worldwide,[48] the shortage of nurses is apparent in both urban and rural regions. Lack of adequate numbers of psychiatric nurses to address clients' mental health care needs can lead to inadequate delivery of treatment processes.

Psychiatric Nursing Treatment Processes

Upon admission to a psychiatric healthcare environment, the holistic assessment is implemented by a nurse. Information about the patient is obtained through observation, interviews, and examination. Family members are especially helpful in situations where the client is unable to provide the information needed or relays un-factual information during the nursing assessment. In the evaluation process, there is both subjective and objective data gathered, including the following:

1. Patient's perception of current symptoms, stressors, or problems
2. Family history
3. Previous hospitalizations
4. Current or past substance use
5. Medical examination: diagnostic investigations, somatic complaints, physical exam
6. Abuse history
7. Spiritual status
8. Mental health examination: thought processes, judgment, awareness, mood and affect, behavior, response to environment, and appearance
9. Coping patterns

The evaluation process is an ongoing practice throughout the client's stay to assist in obtaining the most beneficial specialized interventions and outcomes for each patient.

A nursing diagnosis that addresses both the adaptive and maladaptive health responses and contributing stressors is developed after all the initial data is gathered and evaluated. The diagnosis represents the nurse's clinical judgment. There are three parts to the nursing diagnosis: health problems, contributing factors, and defining characteristics. It is imperative that the defining characteristics are specific and accurate, as they provide the basis for nursing intervention. There can be multiple diagnoses for one patient, and each diagnosis must have measurable, clear, obtainable goals.

Outcome identification is individualized, with each patient assisting in formulating an ultimate goal that influences health outcomes and improves the patient's mental and physical health. In the psychiatric setting, the goals often address behavioral issues and should be developed with client participation. Formulating and clarifying goals with the client and family is an essential part of the nursing treatment, and short-term goals should contribute to the long-term expected outcomes.

Planning involves formulation of the nursing care plan; each nursing diagnosis, short and long-term goals, and interventions are prioritized and written as the nursing process of care. Expected outcomes can be formulated with the evidence-based Nursing Outcomes Classification to obtain the utilization of standardized language, which improves the consistency of terminology, definition, and outcome measures. The nursing care plan needs to be communicated to other members of the healthcare team. Document 3.1 is an example of a mental health nursing care plan.

The plan of care is then implemented. Nursing will continue to assess the client during this phase to ensure that the interventions developed are beneficial in obtaining the desired goals. New nursing diagnoses may need to be implemented as goals are obtained or are found to be unachievable. This process provides a feedback technique for assessing the quality of care provided.

Shortages of nurses to provide mental health care within countries impact the client on many treatment levels, including assessment, planning, outcome identification, and the ability to improve an individual's physical and mental health. Additionally, the delivery of mental health services in a therapeutic manner is essential to recovery processes for clients.

The Therapeutic Relationship

The development of a therapeutic relationship (a fundamental element of health care) is an essential component of providing effective interventions that improve the quality of mental health care. The relationship between the health care worker and the client has to be professional and based on knowledge of the client's history, specific diagnosis, and capacity to heal. A study conducted in 2008 revealed there were nine core elements to developing a therapeutic mental health care relationship:

1. Conveying understanding and empathy
2. Accepting individuality
3. Providing support
4. Being there/being available
5. Being genuine

DOCUMENT 3.1 Nursing Care Plan Example.

NURSING CARE PLAN DEPRESSION

Assessment Data	Nursing Diagnosis	Expected Outcomes (or Planning)	Implementation Nursing Intervention *denotes collaborative interventions	Rationale	Evaluation
• Suicidal ideas or behavior • Slowed mental processes • Disordered thoughts • Feelings of despair, hopelessness, and worthlessness • Guilt • Anhedonia (inability to experience pleasure) • Disorientation • Generalized restlessness or agitation • Sleep disturbances: early awakening, Insomnia, or excessive sleeping • Anger or hostility (may not be overt) • Rumination • Delusions, hallucinations, or other psychotic symptoms • Sexual dysfunction: diminished interest in sexual activity, inability to experience pleasure • Fear of intensity of feelings • Anxiety	• **Ineffective Coping** *Inability to form a valid appraisal of the stressors, inadequate choices of practiced responses, and/or inability to use available resources*	**Immediate** *The client will* • Be free from self-inflicted harm • Engage in reality-based interactions • Be oriented to person, place, and time • Express anger or hostility outwardly in a safe manner **Stabilization** *The client will* • Express feelings directly with congruent verbal and nonverbal messages • Be free from psychotic symptoms • Demonstrate functional level of psychomotor activity **Community** *The client will* • Demonstrate compliance with and knowledge of medications, if any • Demonstrate an increased ability to cope with anxiety, stress, or frustration • Verbalize or demonstrate acceptance of loss or change, if any • Identify a support system in the community	Provide a safe environment for the client. Continually assess the client's potential for suicide. Observe the client closely, especially under the following circumstances: After antidepressant medication begins to raise the client's mood After any sudden dramatic behavioral change (sudden cheerfulness, relief, freedom from guilt, or giving away personal belongings) Unstructured time on the unit Times when the number of staff on the unit is limited	Physical safety of the client is a priority. Many common items and environmental situations may be used by the client in a self-destructive manner. Depressed clients may have a potential for suicide that may or may not be expressed and that may change with time. You must remain aware of this suicide potential at all times. You must be aware of the client's activities at all times when there is a potential for suicide or self-injury: Risk of suicide increases as the client's energy level is increased by medication. These changes may indicate that the client has come to a decision to commit suicide. Risk of suicide increases when the client's time is unstructured. Risk of suicide increases when observation of the client decreases.	

6. Promoting equality
7. Demonstrating respect
8. Maintaining clear boundaries
9. Having self-awareness[49]

Conclusions from this particular study revealed that the core elements can overlap in multiple ways and add to overcoming obstacles by formulating therapeutic relationships within the psychiatric health care spectrum.

The ability of the mental health professional to analyze and adjust approaches to obtain therapeutic outcomes is an essential skill set that develops over time. Professionals beginning their practice in psychiatric settings may need additional supervision and counseling to provide therapeutic care. Some barriers that contribute to difficulties in the development of therapeutic relationships in psychiatric settings are time-related factors, communication barriers, client length of stay, and institutional policies and procedures.

There are many factors that impact the global mental healthcare crisis, but with mental health professionals, there is also the increased level of potential personal harm related to client aggressive behaviors, which, as stated previously, can deter people from choosing this branch of medicine, or motivate mental healthcare workers to quit the mental health profession. Violence is many times exhibited in psychiatric settings, and it is often difficult to predict. An analysis of homicides of mental health care workers by psychiatric patients conducted by George Washington University School of Medicine revealed that the majority of perpetrators of lethal violence were males with the diagnosis of schizophrenia. Studies revealed that 50% to 60% of mental health care workers can expect to be threatened, 30% to 40% can expect to be assaulted, 40% can expect to receive some type of physical injury, and up to 5% can expect to incur serious physical harm. Of the homicides identified in this study, 60.6% were licensed professionals, and 39.4% were technical or case workers.[50]

An *International Journal of Nursing Studies* analysis published in 2020 stated that therapeutic alliance is a core part of the nursing role and key to the attainment of positive outcomes for people using mental health services, but the evidence base for methods to support nursing staff to develop and maintain good therapeutic relationships is poor.[51] In addition to the therapeutic relationship assisting in the development of efficient mental health care services, there must be the utilization of evidence-based care.

Evidence-Based Care

Another obstacle in mental health care is the utilization of evidence-based care. Evidence-based care is defined as the integration of clinical expertise, client values and preferences, and the best research evidence into the decision-making process for patient care. A study conducted in 2018 reveals that evidence-based practice improves the quality of care, patient safety and satisfaction, professional development of mental health care workers, and long-term cost-effectiveness in health care.[52]

The study also identified the barriers to the implementation of evidence-based practices in the mental health setting, including lack of time, skills, and reliable resources; resistance to change; lack of organizational support; and limited interventional studies in the mental health area.[53] Organizations such as SAMHSA have implemented evidence-based practices (EVP) resource centers that contain a collection of scientifically based resources assisting communities and organizations with the implementation of EVP into their treatment modalities.

Using evidence-based mental health care can help decrease liability by ensuring that clinicians are providing the most effective treatments available.[54] This can also help reduce the risk of malpractice claims by ensuring the best practices in the field are being implemented.

Legal and Ethical Dilemmas

There are both ethical and legal dilemmas in the mental health care profession. Ethics, in general, can be referred to as being moral principles and practices. Bioethics is a branch of ethical dilemmas that addresses what is considered right or wrong in the field of medicine or the healthcare profession. The principles of bioethics are nonhierarchical and include a duty to act to benefit patients (beneficence), respecting the client's right to make their own decisions (autonomy), the distribution of resources equally and fairly (justice), maintaining loyalty and commitment to patients with nonintent to create harm or injury (nonmaleficence), and communicating truthfully and honestly (veracity).

Mental health professionals have many roles while assisting in the treatment of clients that can lead to the worker being a moral agent, advocate, and educator for the patient. An example would be that the client has a right to make decisions about their medical treatment, free from controlling influences (coercion or coaxing).

In the instances of mental illness, clients could be easily coerced or make inappropriate decisions with regard to health care practices. A mental health professional, in some circumstances, may need to advocate for the patient and provide education to obtain the best practice outcomes. The WHO has 10 basic principles for mental health care:

1. Promotion of mental health and prevention of mental disorders: Everyone should benefit from the best possible measures to promote their mental well-being and to prevent mental disorders.
2. Access to basic mental healthcare systems: Everyone in need should have access to basic mental health care.

3. Mental health assessments in accordance with internationally accepted principles: Mental health assessments should be made in accordance with internationally accepted medical principles and instruments.
4. Provision of the least restrictive type of mental health: Persons with mental health disorders should be provided with health care that is the least restrictive.
5. Self-determination: Consent is required before any type of interference with a person can occur.
6. Right to be assisted in the exercise of self-determination: In a case where a patient merely experiences difficulties in appreciating the implications of a decision, although not unable to decide, he/she shall benefit from the assistance of a knowledgeable third party of his or her choice.
7. Availability of review procedure: There should be a review procedure available for any decision made by official (judge) or surrogate (representative, e.g., guardian) decision-makers and by health care providers.
8. Automatic periodical review of mechanism: In the case of a decision affecting integrity (treatment) and/or liberty (hospitalization) with a long-lasting impact, there should be an automatic periodical review mechanism.
9. Qualified decision-maker: Decision-makers acting in an official capacity (e.g., judge) or surrogate (consent-giving) capacity (e.g., relative, friend, guardian) shall be qualified to do so.
10. Respect for the rule of law: Decisions should be made in keeping with the body of law in force in the jurisdiction involved and not on another basis nor on an arbitrary basis.[55]

It is imperative that WHO principles are followed globally to deter ongoing improper treatment of patients, as exhibited in Box 3.1. The United States does work to improve mental health care in America through legislation, such as the bill of rights for patients.

BOX 3.1 Guatemala Psychiatric Hospital

A psychiatric hospital in Guatemala is deemed one of the most dangerous mental health institutions in existence. The Federico Mora Hospital houses approximately 340 patients, including many violent and mentally disturbed criminals. The U.S. campaign group Disability Rights International collected evidence on the hospital and released a report in 2012, stating, "Any person with or without a disability detained in this hospital faces immediate risk to his or her life, health, and personal integrity, as well as risk of inhumane and degrading treatment or torture." The report explained that patients were denied medical care, exposed to serious and contagious illnesses and infections, and the issues were compounded by "widespread" sexual abuse—leaving patients at risk of contracting HIV.[56]

Mental Health Systems Act

The 1980 Mental Health Systems Act sets forth a bill of rights for any person admitted to a mental healthcare facility in the United States that includes the following:

- The right to appropriate treatment in a supportive and as nonrestrictive setting as possible.
- The right to individualized treatment and periodic review of such treatment and related services.
- The right to ongoing participation and input, to the extent possible, in the planning of such treatment and reasonable explanation of the state of health, treatment, and objectives, and related matters.
- The right to not receive a course of treatment in the absence of informed, voluntary, written consent, except during an emergency or as legally permitted.
- The right to not participate in involuntary experimentation and to appropriate protection during any such participation.
- The right to nontreatment from restraint or seclusion, except during an emergency.
- The right to confidentiality of and access to medical records.
- The right to be informed of these rights and their exercise without reprisal.[57]

In earlier centuries, there were breaches in many patients' rights that led to alternate regulations being implemented within the industry.

Civil Rights and Tort Laws

Civil rights and tort laws are applicable to the mental health care continuum. Civil rights are the right to be free from discrimination based on protected characteristics (i.e., gender, race, disability, etc.). A violation of civil rights is demonstrated when an individual (or individuals) in certain situations are discriminated against on the basis of protected characteristics. Since some mental illness diagnoses are considered a disability, it would be a breach of civil rights to discriminate against individuals inflicted with a mental condition. The case in Box 3.2 raises many legal and ethical issues in relation to client treatment.

A tort is defined simply as a civil wrong. Tort laws are designed to determine if a person should be held legally liable for an injury (suffering or loss) caused to another human being and the compensation the injured person is entitled to. Torts can be applicable to mental health care in circumstances where health care employees fail to protect the safety of a client/clients. Intentional torts are committed when a health care provider knew or should have known that his/her actions or omissions would result in harm. Negligence torts encompass actions that are unreasonable or unsafe, not following the rules or policies that are developed to prevent harm to others. Strict

BOX 3.2 Connecticut Valley Hospital

The Whiting Forensic Division of Connecticut Valley Hospital in Middleton, Connecticut, had 31 employees suspended and 9 arrested in September 2017 for cruelty to persons and disorderly conduct. Senator Heather Somers stated, "The abuse represents a violation of basic human rights, regardless of the patient's background, and the duration of the maltreatment points to a serious lack of leadership." The state Department of Public Health issued a 102-page inspection report on Whiting, saying as many as 40 staff members "were identified in the video log as being abusive or witnessing abuse" and not reporting it. The report describes employees going into a patient's room, kicking him, throwing food and liquids on him, pulling the sheets over his head—and simply walking out of the room, only to return later to repeat the actions.[58] An updated news release in November 2017 stated that 37 employees at the hospital were implicated in the alleged patient abuse, with 7 being fired and 10 arrested.[59]

liability torts are applicable when harm occurs to a client without proof of direct fault or negligence by a healthcare provider.

In the case of mental illness, it appears that a definitive line that establishes both client and mental health care worker safety is hard to draw due to the client's diagnosis. The mental health cases presented in this book do provide clear data that there is a need to evaluate the mental healthcare system globally and develop and implement a mental health continuum that is beneficial to the safety of those experiencing mental illness and those who provide their care.

BOX 3.3 A Critical Thinking Synopsis—Do You Agree?

The ongoing decline in mental health practitioners adds to increased caseloads for existing practitioners and clients in need of services going without treatment. Worldwide, medical schools are addressing the dynamic by implementing additional incentives to go into this branch of medicine and increasing new residency slots. In the United States, there has been an increase in students going into psychiatry, but the results from this process have yet to be seen.

The same exists with nursing; fewer and fewer individuals are choosing the mental health profession as a career choice, and strategies to curb the crisis have not been met to date, impacting the number of professional nurses available to deliver mental health care globally, thus impacting mental health care recipients.

Strategies implemented by governments have been or are being developed to address the ongoing shortages, but there is no short-term fix for the problem, contributing to the pervasive mental healthcare crisis.

Main Points

1. The goal of mental health treatment is to improve a patient's mental health.
2. In the United States, it is estimated that in 2021, over one third of Americans lived in an area lacking mental health care practitioners.
3. Other countries are experiencing shortages of mental health care practitioners; it is estimated that the number of psychiatrists per population is expected to decrease by 15% by 2030.
4. Most counselors in the United States have stated that they are unable to accept new clients due to an already existing workload.
5. There are also mental health nursing shortages globally; it has been relayed by some individuals who have studied the mental healthcare crisis that a general lack of interest in psychiatric nursing is the major contributing factor to the shortage.
6. The development of a therapeutic relationship (a fundamental element of health care) is an essential component of providing effective interventions that improve the quality of mental health care.
7. Evidence-based care is defined as the integration of clinical expertise, client values and preferences, and the best research evidence into the decision-making process for patient care.
8. There are both ethical and legal dilemmas in the mental health care profession; civil rights and tort laws are applicable to the mental health care continuum.

Notes

1. Jhangiani, Rajiv, PhD (2016), *Introduction to psychology, history of psychology,* Press Books, https://pressbooks.bccampus.ca/kpupsyc1100/chapter/history-of-psychology (accessed August 19, 2023).
2. Cavanaugh, Ray (2015), The founder of modern psychiatry, *History Today,* 65(4), https://www.historytoday.com/archive/founder-modern-psychiatry (accessed August 19, 2023).
3. World Health Organization (2015), *Global health workforce, finances remain low for mental health,* https://www.who.int/news/item/14-07-2025-global-health-workforce-finances-remain-low-for-mental-health/ (accessed August 19, 2023).
4. Statista (2023), *Rate of global mental health workforce in 2020, by type,* https://www.statista.com/ststistics/796082/mental-health-workforce-per-population-rate-worldwide-by-type/ (accessed August 19, 2023).
5. Michas, Frederich (2022), *Psychiatrists: number practicing in Europe 2020, by country,* https://www.statista.com/statistics/554961/psychiatrists-practicing-in-europe (accessed April 26, 2022).
6. Canadian Medical Association (2019), *Psychiatry profile,* Pathway Evaluation Program, https://www.cma.ca/default/files/2019-01/psychiatry-e.pdf (accessed April 26, 2022), pp. 8.

7. USA Facts (2021), *Over one-third of Americans live in areas lacking mental health professionals*, https://wwwusafacts.org/articles/over-one-third-of-americans-live-in-areas-lacking-mental-health-professionals/ (accessed November 23, 2021).

8. USA Facts (2021), *Over one-third of Americans live in areas lacking mental health professionals*, https://wwwusafacts.org/articles/over-one-third-of-americans-live-in-areas-lacking-mental-health-professionals/ (accessed November 23, 2021).

9. Smith, Andy (2021), Shortage of psychiatrists and mental health providers projected to rise, *Healthcare Solutions*, https://insynchcs.com/blog/rising-shortage-mental-health-professionals (accessed November 23, 2021).

10. Smith, Andy (2021), Shortage of psychiatrists and mental health providers projected to rise, *Healthcare Solutions*, https://insynchcs.com/blog/rising-shortage-mental-health-professionals (accessed November 23, 2021).

11. U.S. Bureau of Labor Statistics (2023), *Occupational employment and wages, May 2022: Psychiatrists*, https://www.bls.gov/oes/current/oes193039.htm#nat (accessed August 19, 2023).

12. Zippia (2023), *Clinical psychologist demographics and statistics in the U.S.*, https://www.zippia,com/clinical-psychologist-jobs-demographics/ (accessed August 19, 2023).

13. Bureau of Labor Statistics, U.S. Department of Labor (2022), *Occupational outlook handbook, psychologists*, https://www.bls.gov/ooh/life-physical-and-social-science/psychologists.htm (accessed August 19, 2023).

14. Weiner, Stacey (2022), *A growing psychiatrist shortage and an enormous demand for mental health services*, Association of American Medical Colleges, https://www.aamc.org/news/growing-psychiatrist-shortage-enormous-demand-mental-health-services (accessed August 19, 2023).

15. United States Government Accountability Office (2022), *Behavioral health, available workforce information and federal actions to help recruit and retain providers*, https://www.gao.gov/products/gao-23-105250 (accessed August 19, 2023), pp. 16, 17.

16. Moran, Mark (2021), *Psychiatry residency match numbers climb again after unprecedented year in medical education, Psychiatric News*, American Psychiatric Association, https://doi.org/10.1176/appi.pn.2021.5.27 (accessed August 19, 2023).

17. Weiner, Stacey (2022), *A growing psychiatrist shortage and an enormous demand for mental health services*, Association of American Medical Colleges, https://www.aamc.org/news/growing-psychiatrist-shortage-enormous-demand-mental-health-services (accessed August 19, 2023).

18. Ontario Psychiatric Association (2019), *Ontario needs psychiatrists*, https://www.eopa.ca/sites/default/uploads/files/ontario-needs-psychiatrists/2018.pdf (accessed November 27, 2021), pp. 1–10.

19. Ontario Psychiatric Association (2019), *Ontario needs psychiatrists*, https://www.eopa.ca/sites/default/uploads/files/ontario-needs-psychiatrists/2018.pdf (accessed November 27, 2021), pp. 1–10.

20. Rimmer, Abi (2021), Mental health: Staff shortages are causing distressing long waits for treatment, college warns, *BMJ*, 375:n2439, https://doi.org/10.1136/bmj.n2439 (accessed November 27, 2021).

21. Australian Medical Association (2021), *AMA response to National Mental Health Workforce Strategy consultation*, https://www.ama.com.au/articles/ama-response-to-national-

mental-health-workforce-strategy-consultation/draft (accessed November 27, 2021). pp. 1–6.

22. Weiner, Stacey (2022), *A growing psychiatrist shortage and an enormous demand for mental health services*, Association of American Medical Colleges, https://www.aamc.org/news/growing-psychiatrist-shortage-enormous-demand-mental-health-services (accessed August 19, 2023).
23. Weinburg, Tessa (2021), Mental health staffing shortages limit access to patient care, *The Missouri Independent*, https://newstribune.com/news/2021/nov/05/Mental-health-staff-ing-shortages-limit-access-to-p/#:~:text=A%20staffing%20crisis%20across%20state-run%20mental%20health%20facilities,officials%20told%20the%20Mental%20Health%20Commis-sion%20on%20Thursday (accessed December 5, 2022).
24. Bureau of Labor Statistics, U.S. Department of Labor (2023), *Occupational outlook handbook, psychologists*, https://www.bls.ooh/gov/healthcare/psychiatric-technicians-and-aids.htm (accessed August 19, 2023).
25. Zippa (2022), *Mental health counselor demographics and statistics in the US*, The Career Expert, https://www.zippa.com/mental-health-counselor-jobs/demographics/ (accessed December 5, 2022).
26. U.S. Bureau of Labor Statistics (2021), *Occupational employment and wages, May 2021: Marriage and family therapists*, https://www.bls.gov/ooh/community-and-social-service/marriage-and-family-therapists.htm#:~:text=The%20median%20annual%20wage%20for%20marriage%20and%20family,much%20faster%20than%20the%20average%20for%20all%20occupations (accessed December 5, 2022).
27. Zippa (2022), *Licensed social worker demographics and statistics in the US*, The Career Expert, https://www.zippa.com/licensed-social-worker-jobs/demographics/. (accessed December 5, 2022).
28. Centers for Disease Control and Prevention (2021), *About mental health*, https://www.cdc.gov/mentalhealth/learn/index.htm (accessed December 5, 2022).
29. Rural Health Information Hub (2022), *Health professional shortage areas: Mental health by county, 2022*, https://www.rural healthinfo.org/charts/7 (accessed December 5, 2022).
30. Wikipedia, *Psychiatric and mental health nursing*, http://en.wikipedia.org/wiki/psychiat-ric_and_mental_health_nursing (accessed November 26, 2017).
31. Wikipedia, *Psychiatric and mental health nursing*, http://en.wikipedia.org/wiki/psychiatric_and_mental_health_nursing (accessed November 26, 2017).
32. Zauszniewski, A.J. PhD, et al. (2012). A decade of published evidence for psychiatric and mental health nursing interventions, *OJIN: The Online Journal of Issues in Nursing*,17(3), 8, https://pubmed.ncb.nlm.nih.gov/23036061 (accessed November 5, 2019).
33. Zauszniewski, A.J. PhD, et al. (2012), A decade of published evidence for psychiatric and mental health nursing interventions, *OJIN: The Online Journal of Issues in Nursing*,17(3), 8, https://pubmed.ncb.nlm.nih.gov/23036061. (accessed November 5, 2019).
34. Zauszniewski, A.J. PhD, et al. (2012), A decade of published evidence for psychiatric and mental health nursing interventions, *OJIN: The Online Journal of Issues in Nursing*, 17(3), 8, https://pubmed.ncb.nlm.nih.gov/23036061. (accessed November 5, 2019).
35. Wikipedia, *Psychiatric and mental health nursing*, http://en.wikipedia.org/wiki/psychiatric_and_mental_health_nursing (accessed November 26, 2017).

36. Wikipedia, *Psychiatric and mental health nursing,* http://en.wikipedia.org/wiki/psychiatric_and_mental_health_nursing (accessed November 26, 2017).

37. eGyanKosh (2017), *Historical development of psychiatric nursing,* https://www.egyankosh.ac.in/bitstream/123456789/31553/1/unit-1.pdf (accessed January 5, 2022), pp. 9.

38. Jensen, Phyllis (2015), Nursing, *The Canadian Encyclopedia,* https://www.thecanadianencyclopedia.ca/en/article/nursing (accessed January 5, 2022).

39. Stegge, GJ (2004), Psychiatric training of nurses in the Netherlands since 1883, *Gewina,* 27(2), https://www.pubmed.ncbi.nlm..nih.gov/15359463/. (accessed January 5, 2022), pp.78–99.

40. Zippia (2023), *Psychiatric nurse practitioner demographics and statistics in the US,* https://www.zippia.com/psychiatric-nurse-practitioner-jobs-demographics/ (accessed August 19, 2023).

41. Murez, Cara (2022), Nurse practitioners are filling the gap in U.S. psychiatric care, *U.S. News,* https://www.usnews.com/news/health-news/articles/2022-09-08/nurse-practitioners-are-filling-the-gap-in-u-s-psychiatric-care (accessed August 19, 2023).

42. Murez, Cara (2022), Nurse practitioners are filling the gap in U.S. psychiatric care, *U.S. News,* https://www.usnews.com/news/health-news/articles/2022-09-08/nurse-practitioners-are-filling-the-gap-in-u-s-psychiatric-care (accessed August 19, 2023).

43. Bureau of Labor Statistics, U.S. Department of Labor (2021), *Occupational employment and wage statistics,* https://www.bls.gov/oes/current/oes291141.htm (accessed September 20, 2022).

44. Michas, Frederic (2022), *Global mental health workforce rate per 100,000 population by type 2020,* Statista, https://www.staista.Com/statistics/796082/mental-health-workforce-per-popilation-rate-worldwide-by-type (accessed December 6, 2022).

45. Registered Psychiatric Nurse Regulators in Canada (2022), *Registered psychiatric nursing in Canada,* https://rpnc.ca/registered-psychiatric-nursing-canada#:~:text=There%20are%20over%206%2C000%20Registered%20Psychiatric%20Nurses%20%28RPNs%29,client-centered%20services%20to%20individuals%2C%20families%2C%20groups%20and%20communities (accessed December 9, 2022).

46. World Health Organization (2019), *Mental health workers data by country,* https://apps.who.int/gho/data/view.main. HWF11v,(accessed December 9, 2022).

47. Michas, Frederic (2022), *Total number of mental health nurses in the NHS Hospitals and Community Health Service (HCHS) workforce in England from 2009 to 2021,* Statista, https://www.statista.com/statistics/679563/number-of-mental-health-nurses-inhs-workforce-england/#:~:text=The%20number%20of%20mental%20health%20nurses%20had%20been,%28HCHS%29%20workforce%20in%20England%20from%202009%20to%202021%2A (accessed December 9, 2022).

48. World Health Organization (2020), *World mental health day: an opportunity to kick-start a massive scale-up in investment in mental health,* https://www.who.int/news/item/27-08-2020-world-mental-health-day-an-opportunity-to-kick-start-a-massive-investment-in-mental-health (accessed May 2, 2022).

49. Dziopa, F. and Ahern, K. (2008), What makes a quality therapeutic relationship in psychiatric/mental health nursing: A review of the research literature, *The Internet Journal of Advanced Nursing Practice,* 10(1), https://www.ispub.com/IJANP/10/1/7218 (accessed February 6, 2022).

50. Knable, Michael, DO (2017), *Homicides of mental health workers by patients*, George Washington University School of Medicine, https://mentalillnesspolicy.org/wp-content/homicidementalhealthworkers.pdf (accessed December 12, 2018).

51. Hartley, Samantha, et al. (2020), Effective nurse-patient relationships in mental health care: A systematic review of interventions to improve the therapeutic alliance, *Int J Nurs Stud*, (102), https://ncbi.nlm.gov/pmc/articles/PMC7026691/ (accessed August 19, 2023).

52. Karki, Asmita (2018), *Implementation of evidence-based care in mental health nursing: Barriers and strategies*, https://www.thesus.fi/bitstream/handle/10024/166757/asmita%20-thesis.pdf?sequence=2 (accessed February 6, 2022), pp. 2.

53. Karki, Asmita (2018), *Implementation of evidence-based care in mental health nursing: Barriers and strategies*, https://www.thesus.fi/bitstream/handle/10024/166757/asmita%20-thesis.pdf?sequence=2 (accessed February 6, 2022), pp. 2.

54. Geddes, John, et al. (1998), Evidence-based practice in mental health, *BMJ*,1(1), https://mentalhealth.bmj.com/content/1/1/4 (accessed August 19, 2023), pp. 4–5.

55. World Health Organization, (1996), *Mental health care law: Ten basic principles*, Division of Mental Health and Prevention of Substance Abuse, https://apps.who.int/iris/bitstream/handle/10665/63624/WHO_MNH_MND_96.9.pdf?sequence=1&isAllowed=y (accessed December 7, 2017), pp.1–8.

56. Rogers, Chris (2014), *Inside the world's most dangerous hospital*, BBC News, www.bbc.com/news/magazine-30293880 (accessed December 7, 2017).

57. S.1177-Mental Health Systems Act. 96th Congress (1979–1980), https://www.congress.gov/bill/96th-congress/senate-bill/1177 (accessed December 10, 2017).

58. Goslee, Kaitlin (2017), *Public health committee drills hospital administrator over alleged patient abuse*, FOX 61 news, https://www.fox61.com/article/news/local/outreach/awareness-months/public-hearing-monday-morning-on-alleged-abuse (accessed December 7, 2017).

59. Kovner, Josk (2017), 9 arrested so far in patient abuse scandal at Whiting Forensic; 31 workers were suspended, *Hartford Courant*, https://www.courat.com/news/connecticut/hc-whiting-forensic-patient-abuse-arrests-0906-2017-0905-story.html (accessed December 7, 2017).

Credits

Fig. 3.1: Copyright © by Microsoft. Reprinted with permission.
Fig. 3.2a: Data Source: https://www.statista.com/statistics/554961/psychiatrists-practising-in-europe.
Fig. 3.2b: Data Source: https://www.cma.ca/sites/default/files/2019-01/psychiatry-e.pdf.

CHAPTER 4

Substance Use Disorder and Treatment Programs

The main objective of this chapter is for the reader to have a deeper insight into comorbidity, factors related to a dual diagnosis, how deinstitutionalization has impacted substance misuse, and recommended treatment options for successful recovery.

Substance misuse is a global problem; discussions in this chapter will assist in understanding the scope of the dilemma through the presentation of worldwide statistics, explanations on how mental illness and substance misuse are comorbid diseases that can exacerbate each other, presented evidence on the harmful effects of many substances, and elaborations on the treatment options for substance misuse. There are some other aspects to consider with substance misuse and how it relates to the mental healthcare crisis, such as the lack of provision of comorbid treatment, the statistics on how many people actually receive treatment, and how substance misuse can compound ongoing mental and physical health adversities, contributing to increased healthcare costs.

Deinstitutionalization may also be a factor in increased illegal drug utilization, as those inflicted with mental disease attempt to self-medicate. In communities without established adequate mental health services and housing, there could be a lack of availability for individuals to obtain assessment and treatment in mental health cases. Because of this lack of adequate availability of mental health practitioners and/or services, individuals experiencing mental conditions may misuse illicit drugs to attempt to manage their symptomatology. Reasons for the increased vulnerability to the problematic use of substances in mental illness are the enhancement of rewarding effects, reduced awareness of the illicit drug's negative effects, and/or alleviation of the unpleasant symptoms of a mental condition or the side effects of medication used to treat it.[1]

It is also widely believed that individuals experiencing mental conditions attempt to self-medicate with illicit drug utilization when experiencing subclinical symptomatology. There are many studies that have been conducted and are still being conducted encompassing the correlation between the two diagnoses, with some of the findings revealing the following:

- Undiagnosed mental illness can lead to substance misuse because of the individual attempting to self-medicate the symptoms of the psychiatric condition.
- Diagnosed psychiatric clients often take medications that have unpleasant side effects. Clients often use illicit substances to alleviate these side effects.
- A few illicit drugs can cause mental illness after years of chronic misuse.
- Individuals who are at risk for mental illness increase that risk when they chronically misuse illicit substances.
- Heavy illicit drug utilization during adolescent years can lead to mental illness later in life.[2]

Comorbidity

The term comorbidity is defined as the presence of two or more diagnoses in a person, which can occur simultaneously or subsequently. In the United States, approximately 9.5 million individuals have both a mental illness and a substance use problem.[3] It was estimated that 49.4% of adults with an SMI and 6.7% of adults with any mental illness used illegal drugs in 2018.[4] In 2021, it was estimated that illicit drug use was at 21% for any mental illness and 31.4% for an SMI in the United States.[5]

According to SAMHSA, in 2023, 13.5% of young adults aged 18 to 25 had both a substance use disorder (SUD) and any mental illness in 2021.[6] The author's experience while employed as a psychiatric nurse substantiates SAMHSA's percentages. There were individuals in their 20s admitted to the psychiatric institution for drug-induced psychosis, and for some of the patients, the damage was permanent.

In the United Kingdom, nearly two thirds (63%, or 82,613) of adults starting substance use treatment in 2021 said they had a mental health treatment need. This is part of a trend of rising numbers over the previous 2 years (from 53% in 2018 to 2019).[7] Australian Government statistics from the National Drug Strategy Household Survey (NDSHS) revealed that, in 2019, compared with people without mental health conditions, people with a mental health condition were 1.7 times as likely to have recently used any illicit drug (26% compared with 15.2%).[8]

A 2012 Canadian Community Health Survey—Mental Health estimated that 282,000 Canadians experienced a mental health condition and SUD concurrently in the year previous to the survey.[9] In 2019, it was estimated that the percentage of Canadians with a mental illness who also have a substance use problem was 20%.[10] Another study that examined European countries revealed that lifetime comorbidity differed by country—35% in the United Kingdom, 21% in Germany, and 19% in France.[11]

Substance Use Disorder

Substance misuse is considered to be a mental illness in and of itself because it alters brain functionality, disrupting an individual's normal hierarchy of needs and desires. A substance misuser will be more focused on procuring and using illegal substances, generating compulsive behaviors that occur despite the consequences in their life. SUD is defined as a chronic brain disease that causes compulsive substance use despite harmful consequences with regard to health, finances, relationships, and careers.

The *DSM-5-TR* (*Diagnostic and Statistical Manual of Mental Disorders, Fifth Edition, Text Revision*) identifies one diagnosis for drug use, SUD, which combines the abuse and disorder diagnosis from previous years and requires 2 criteria out of 11 in a 12-month period for a diagnosis.[12] There are many substances that individuals can misuse; for this discussion, we will examine a few of the most widely used chemicals available in society.

Alcohol

Alcohol is a legal drug that can produce dangerous effects with higher amounts of consumption. Excessive alcohol consumption is a leading factor in serious injury and accidental death. Increased alcohol utilization can lead to alcohol use disorder (AUD), which also can carry a genetic trait and is associated with depression. One hypothesis suggests that individuals with anxiety disorders use alcohol as a tension-reduction mechanism, but this theory has not been validated by many researchers.

A study conducted in Brazil (2013) revealed, "The association between substance use, coping strategies, and symptoms of stress seems to be more important for men than for women. In the possibility of reducing tension, stress seems to be a predictor of increased consumption only for men with positive expectations."[13]

Over the past ten years, rates of AUDs have increased in women by 84%, closing the gap between the genders with the current weighted rate at 9% for adult women and 16.7% for adult men.[14] Including both binge and heavy alcohol users, the totality in the United States (2020) encompassed 138.5 million individuals.[15] Figure 4.1 portrays the number of individuals (data by millions) with AUDs by region.

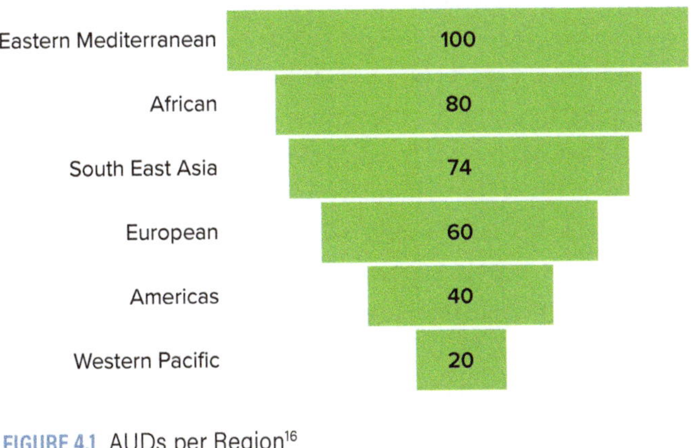

FIGURE 4.1 AUDs per Region[16]

An individual diagnosed with AUD needs inpatient treatment under the supervision of a physician to manage the substance withdrawal. Early treatment is considered to be more effective rather than after the illness has progressed for an extended period of years. A crisis intervention modality in detoxification units in psychiatric hospitals has included five-point leather restraint utilization, as illustrated in Box 4.1.

BOX 4.1 Vermont State Hospital

The Department of Justice reported in July of 2005 that the Vermont State Hospital "consistently uses seclusion and restraint as an intervention of first resort and often uses seclusion/restraint for the convenience of staff and/or as initial punishment." And "over 90% of restraint incidents in Vermont State Hospital involve strapping patients to a bed in five-point restraints in a seclusion room—the most restrictive and dangerous form of intervention."[17]

AUD has serious impacts on an individual's health, including liver damage, heart disease, impotence, high blood pressure, infertility, learning and memory problems, dementia, premature aging, depression and anxiety. Nearly 95,000 people die from alcohol-related causes annually, making it the third preventable leading cause of death in the United States.[18] In 2019, alcohol use accounted for 2.07 million deaths of males and 374,000 deaths of females globally.[19] In 2022, it was estimated that alcohol contributes to around 3 million deaths worldwide per year.[20]

Marijuana

According to the United Nations, 200 million people around the world use marijuana, more than 3.9% of the planet's population.[21] The legalization of marijuana in some American states has been a controversial issue for the medical profession. Marijuana utilization is associated with short-term memory loss, accelerated heart rate, increased blood pressure, difficulty concentrating and processing information, lapsed judgment, and problems encompassing perception associated with motor skills. Long-term utilization of marijuana can lead to increased ambition loss and an inability to function effectively. In Figure 4.2, percentages of marijuana utilization (based on estimates from 113 countries) are provided for several countries.

Several studies have been conducted with regard to marijuana; results revealed that adolescents who carry the genetic factor (catechol-O-methyltransferase, Val variant) are more likely to develop schizophreniform disorder as they progress into their adult lives if these individuals are exposed to cannabis utilization.[23] Recent research revealed that people who use marijuana and carry a specific variant of the AKT1 gene, which codes for an enzyme that affects dopamine signaling, are at increased risk of developing psychosis.[24]

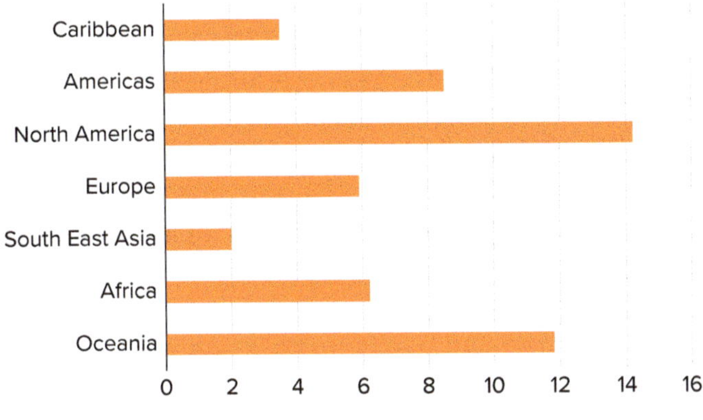

FIGURE 4.2 Percentage of Marijuana Use[22]

Marijuana contains more than 400 known chemicals; the main ingredient that affects the mind is THC (tetrahydrocannabinol).[25] THC levels in the hemp plant have increased over the years; they were 1% in the 1970s, 5% in 1997, 10% in 2008, 12% in 2010, and 20% THC in 2015.[26] A recent study in 2020 concluded that recreational marijuana can contain THC up to 21.5%.[27] THC stays in the body for weeks and possibly months after the drug is used, depending on length and intensity, damaging the immune system and exposing the body to cancer-causing agents for prolonged periods of time. Benzopyrene is the chemical in tobacco that causes lung cancer. An average marijuana cigarette contains nearly 50% more benzopyrene than a tobacco cigarette. An average marijuana cigarette contains 30 nanograms of this carcinogen compared to 21 nanograms in an average tobacco cigarette.[28]

Marijuana and some of its compounds influence the immune system and affect the body's ability to resist viruses, bacteria, fungi, and protozoa, and decrease the body's antitumor activities. Marijuana has the potential to alter the backup safeguards of the immune system because it affects diverse types of cells in the body. This could compromise the immune system's ability to screen out cancer cells and eliminate infection.[29]

In regards to medical marijuana, the FDA has approved one plant-based marijuana drug and two medications made from synthetic chemicals that mimic the actions and effects of THC. These medications are only available with a prescription from a licensed healthcare provider: Epidiolex contains purified CBD from the marijuana plant. The drug is approved for treating seizures associated with two rare and severe forms of epilepsy as well as seizures associated with a rare genetic disorder. Dronabinol and nabilone are made from lab-created chemicals that act like THC by turning on cannabis receptors in the brain. These two medications are used to treat nausea in patients with cancer who are undergoing chemotherapy treatment and to increase appetite in individuals with AIDS who do not feel like eating.[30]

Stimulants/Sedatives

Stimulants include substances such as cocaine, crack, and amphetamines. These chemicals provide the user with an illusion of enhanced power and energy for a temporary period, which then can transpire into depression and potentially violent or paranoid behaviors. Cocaine is the second most used illegal drug in the United States.[31] In Figure 4.3, the global (based on estimates from 84 countries) percentage of cocaine utilization is portrayed.

Colombia is one of the leading producers and traffickers of cocaine. Colombia and the United States reached an agreement in 2018 to obtain a 50% reduction in cocaine production and cultivation of raw material cocoa by 2023.[33] In 2018, almost 4% of 12th graders admitted to having used cocaine at least once in their lives.[34]

It has been suggested that individuals who are cocaine dependent may use the drug to alleviate depression. Long-term amphetamine utilization may result in psychosis with symptoms that can include paranoid delusions and hallucinations. In 2020, a national survey on drug utilization and health study revealed that 2.6 million individuals had used methamphetamines in the past year.[35]

Sedatives are used to relieve anxiety and promote sleep. Harmful effects can occur when taken in excess or without a physician's supervision. There can also be serious paradoxical complications that can occur in conjunction with sedative utilization that can lead to unexpected results, including depression, suicidal tendencies, phobias, aggression, violent behavior, and symptoms sometimes misdiagnosed as psychosis. Combining alcohol and sedatives is a dangerous combination since alcohol slows brain function and depresses respiration.

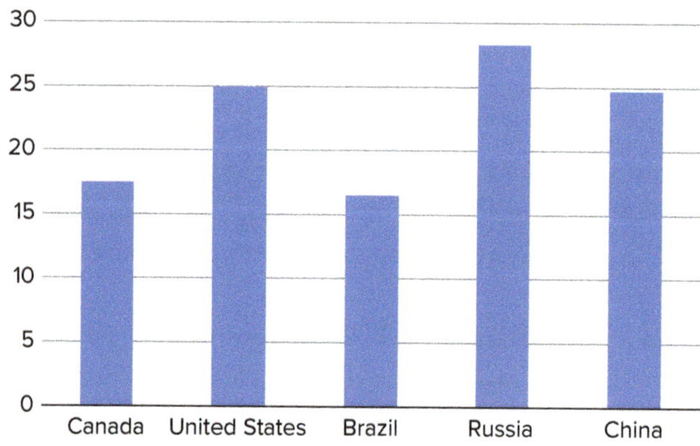

FIGURE 4.3 Percentage Global Cocaine Use[32]

Opioids

Opioids are a class of drugs that include the illegal drug heroin, synthetic opioids such as fentanyl, and pain relievers available by prescription, such as oxycodone, hydrocodone, codeine, morphine, and many others. Overdoses in the U.S. involving opioids killed more than 80,000 people in 2021, and nearly 88% of those deaths involved synthetic opioids.[36] In the United States, over 10 million people abuse opioids every year.[37] It is also estimated that 80% of heroin users have used prescription opioids as well.[38] Figure 4.4 illustrates global opioid rates per million.

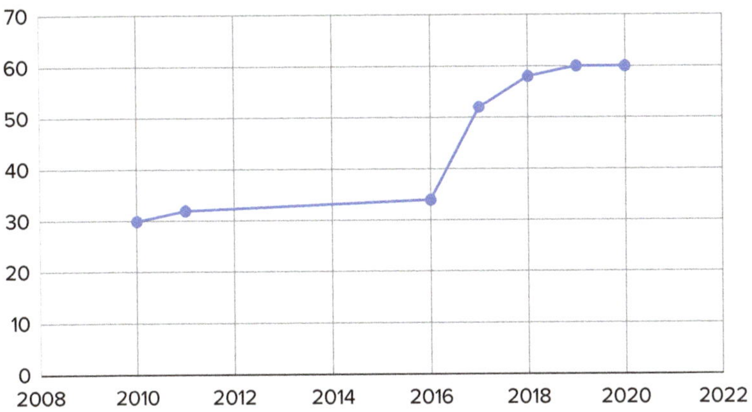

FIGURE 4.4 Global Opioid Utilization Rates[39]

A 2021 analysis of 73 countries revealed the global opioid consumption rate declined by 30% between 2009 and 2019. The reduction in global consumption was primarily driven by decreased opioid consumption in the United States and Germany. In 2009, Germany had the highest consumption rate, followed by the United States and Canada. The consumption rate declined in Germany, the United States, and Canada from 2009 to 2019. In 2019, these three countries were still among those with the highest consumption rates in the world, but the United Kingdom had the highest rate.[40] Worldwide, about 0.5 million deaths annually are attributable to drug use. More than 70% of these deaths are related to opioids, with more than 30% of those deaths caused by overdose.[41]

Inhalants

These products produce mind-altering effects when sniffed or "huffed" and include glue, paint thinners, and lighter fluid. Long-term abuse can result in permanent damage to the nervous system. Inhalants are the fourth most abused substance, and over 2.6 million children between the ages of 12 to 17 use an inhalant each year to get high.[42] Short-term effects from the utilization of inhalants include slurred speech, inability to coordinate movement, hallucinations, delusions, hostility, apathy, impaired judgment, and a drunk or dazed appearance. Over a long period of utilization, inhalant users will display disorientation, depression, irritability, memory impairment, and diminished intelligence.

Nicotine

It is believed that tobacco products have addictive properties as severe as heroin. Approximately 40% of all cigarettes smoked are consumed by adults diagnosed with a mental illness.[43] It is suggested that 70% to 80% of schizophrenic clients use nicotine; researchers report that nicotine may assist schizophrenics in counteracting psychotic symptoms by increasing positive symptom intensity, dealing with social stigma, and alleviating side effects of medications.[44] Percentages of nicotine utilization are exhibited in Figure 4.5.

In the United States, the top cause of preventable deaths is nicotine addiction. The CDC reports that cigarette smoking results in more than 480,00 premature deaths in the United States each year, approximately one in every five deaths.[46]

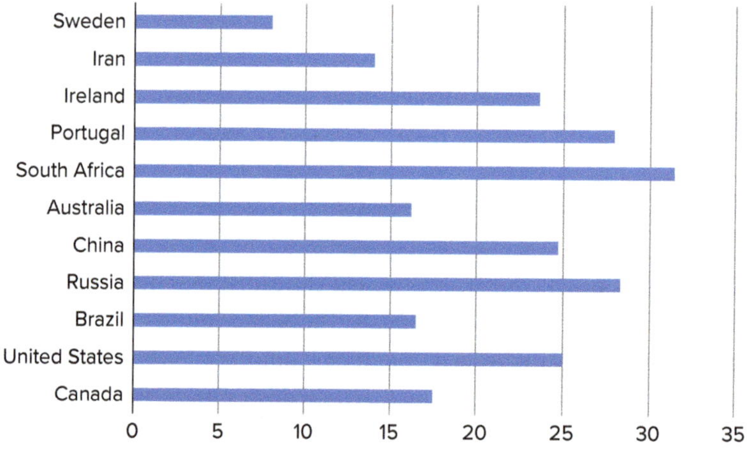

FIGURE 4.5 Nicotine Utilization[45]

Hallucinogens

Ecstasy, PCP (phencyclidine or angel dust), Ketamine, DXM (dextromethorphan), LSD (lysergic acid diethylamide) and DMT (dimethyltryptamine) are chemicals that generate hallucinations (profound distortions in a person's perceptions of reality) and feelings of euphoria. These drugs contain chemicals that are closely related to the chemical structures of serotonin and act as neurotransmitter mimics, thus generating their effects by disrupting the neurotransmission and interaction of brain cells.[47]

In 2020, among people aged 12 to 17 in the United States, 370,000 individuals used hallucinogens in the past year.[48] It was also identified that 7.1 million individuals aged 12 or older used hallucinogens in 2020.[49] In 2022, among U.S. adults aged 19 to 30, 8% reported past-year use of hallucinogens, significantly higher than 5 years ago (5% in 2017) and 10 years ago (3% in 2012).[50] And past-year hallucinogen use reached a historically high prevalence among U.S. adults 35 to 50 years old, reported by 4%

in 2022. The prevalence reported in 2022 was also a substantial increase compared to the year before (2% in 2021).[51]

Hallucinogen utilization in other countries is as follows: Slovakia (males 1.6%/females 0.1%), Poland (males 2.6%/females 0.2%), Czechia (males 2.9%/females 1%), Germany (males 3.4%/females 1.7%), United Kingdom (males 7.6%/females 2.8%).[52]

Major effects identified as being associated with the utilization of hallucinogens are rapid, intense mood swings, increased heart rate and blood pressure, and a high potential for convulsions and seizures. These side effects can vary based on the amount of drug ingested, an individual's personality, mood, and expectations, and whether the individual is alone or with a group.

John Hopkins Center for Psychedelic and Consciousness Research conducts studies on how psychedelics affect behavior, mood, cognition, brain function, and biological markers of health. The institution is expanding studies to explore the effectiveness of psilocybin as therapy for opioid addiction, Alzheimer's disease, post-traumatic stress disorder, Lyme disease syndrome, anorexia nervosa, and alcohol use with major depressive disorder. A recent 2021 article published in the *Harm Reduction Journal, Ethical and Legal Issues in Psychedelic Harm Reduction and Integration Therapy,* explores this dynamic, relaying that recent clinical trials have demonstrated strong evidence of therapeutic benefits.

Comorbidity Common Factors

Both substance misuse and mental illness have hereditary factors, making some individuals more susceptible to both during their lifetime. It has been suggested that genetics, brain neurotransmitter functionality, and environmental factors can contribute to the development of a dual diagnosis. It is estimated that between 40% and 60% of probabilities for drug addiction are related to genetic factors involving both complex factors among multiple genes and genetic factors with environmental influences.[53] Human genomes can act directly or indirectly, and several genetic pairs have been linked to the development of SUD and mental illness.[54] Document 4.1 demonstrates hereditary factors encompassing psychiatric admission processes in 1906.

Certain mental conditions are also more likely to misuse substances, such as antisocial personality disorder, bipolar disorder, depression, anxiety disorders, and post-traumatic stress disorder. Both SUD and mental illness can be caused by overlapping factors such as brain deficits, genetic traits, and early (adverse childhood experiences (ACE)) exposure to stress or trauma.

The neurotransmitter dopamine is altered by addictive substances and is also involved in mental illnesses such as depression and schizophrenia. Alteration of dopamine pathways is associated with environmental factors that generate stress, which is a risk factor for mental conditions, providing one neurobiological link between SUD and other mental illnesses.[55]

DOCUMENT 4.1 1906 Report, "State Hospital Insane" Hereditary Tendencies. Nebraska Literary Commission. The Atrium, 1200 N Street, Suite 120, Lincoln, Nebraska 68508-2023.

HOSPITAL FOR INSANE, INGLESIDE
HEREDITARY TENDENCIES OF PATIENTS.

Admitted during the Biennial Period ending November 30th, 1906.

	Males	Females	Totals
Aunt Insane	1	0	1
Aunts (two) Insane and Father a Dipsomaniac	0	1	1
Brother Insane	3	2	5
Brothers (two) and Sister Insane	1	0	1
Brother and Uncle Insane	0	1	1
Brother Insane and Father a Dipsomaniac	0	1	1
Cousin Insane	1	0	1
Father Epileptic	1	0	1
Father Insane	5	0	5
Father a Dipsomaniac	5	1	6
Father and Brother Insane	1	0	1
Father Suicided	1	0	1
Grandmother Insane	2	0	2
Mother's Aunt Insane	0	1	1
Mother Insane	6	2	8
Mother and Sister Insane	1	0	1
Mother, Sister, Cousin and Mother's Father Insane	0	1	1
Mother and Uncle Insane	1	0	1
Nephew Insane	1	0	1
Sister Insane	8	1	9
Sister Epileptic	1	0	1
Sister and Aunt Insane	0	1	1
Uncle Insane	5	1	6
Uncle Epileptic	1	0	1
Uncle and Cousin Insane	2	0	2
Intemperate, Insane and Epileptic Ancestry	0	1	1
None	53	6	59
Unknown	63	15	78
Totals	**163**	**35**	**198**

Nebraska Library Commission, Ninth Biennial Report of the State Hospital for Insane at Ingleside, Nebraska to the Governor, 1906.

Overlapping of brain region functionality involved in both substance addiction and other mental disorders can have causative effects on each other. Drug addiction developing first may alter brain structure and function, increasing the propensity for the development of another mental condition, and a mental illness developing first generates changes in brain activity, increasing the vulnerability to substance use addiction.[56]

Again, environmental factors are also a contributing element to the development of comorbidity. Parental psychiatric illness, domestic abuse, and a family history of substance misuse are all social/environmental factors that can increase the probability of an apparent dual diagnosis of mental conditions. Also, comorbidity was significantly more of a probability, encompassing the development of psychiatric conditions in clients with early age of first utilization of any drug.

The National Center for Drug Abuse Statistics reported a key finding of increased drug utilization of 61% from 2016 to 2020 among eighth graders in America.[57] Among adults aged 18 or older in 2020 with past-year substance misuse, the percentage of adults with co-occurring mental illness in the past year increased from (8.1 million people) to 17 million people.[58] A lifetime psychiatric condition was identified in approximately half of the comorbid population evaluated in some of these studies. These statistics of comorbidity are evidence of how widespread substance misuse and mental illness are in the United States, and other countries have similar statistics. This substantiates how important the mental health systems for treatment are in attempts to alleviate the mental healthcare crisis.

Treatment

It is believed that only approximately 7.8% of clients attain treatment for both issues. Approximately half of the individuals (51.4%) with a dual diagnosis (comorbidity) do not obtain treatment for either disorder.[59] The first priority in a dual diagnosis case is stabilizing the client through detoxification, removing the illicit substances from the body and managing withdrawal symptoms. Mental illness and SUD both require treatment for a successful recovery to be obtained.

The Joint Committee on Administrative Rules, Administrative Code states SUD treatment shall be offered in varying degrees of intensity based on the level of care in which the patient is placed and the subsequent treatment plan developed for that patient. Patient placement criteria are identified as follows:

- Level 0.5 Early Intervention: Considered subclinical or pretreatment and is designed to explore and address problems or risk factors that appear to be related to substance use and to assist the individual in recognizing the harmful consequences of inappropriate substance use.
- Level 1 Outpatient: Nonresidential substance misuse treatment consisting of face-to-face clinical services. Regularly scheduled sessions that average less than 9 hours per week.

- Level II Intensive Outpatient/Partial Hospitalization: Nonresidential substance use treatment consisting of face-to-face clinical services. Regularly scheduled sessions that are at a minimum of 9 hours per week.
- Level III Inpatient Subacute/Residential: Includes a planned regimen of clinical services for a minimum of 25 hours per week. Staff available on duty 24 hours per day, 7 days per week.
- Level IV Medically Managed Intensive Inpatient: Requires 24-hour medically directed evaluation, care and treatment, and a physician sees the patient daily. Staff available on duty 24 hours per day, 7 days per week.[60]

Scientific research conducted on the treatment of comorbidity reveals that the medical team should treat both diagnoses concurrently. Even when the comorbidities do not occur simultaneously, research demonstrates that psychiatric conditions increase the vulnerability to substance use, and substance use constitutes a risk factor for subsequent mental illness. As stated previously, individuals identified as misusing substances generally will initiate a detoxification and medically managed withdrawal process. This process alone does not address the psychological, social and behavioral problems associated with SUD and will not produce full recovery used independently.

Unfortunately, many individuals inflicted with SUD are in denial of their problem. Plus, SUD is a chronic illness, and these individuals are prone to relapse. The treatment modality should combine medications, individual/group/family therapy, and behavioral therapies. Clinicians and researchers both agree that pharmacological and behavioral therapies, used concurrently, lead to better outcomes for clients with comorbid disorders.[61] There is also some research that demonstrates the utilization of dually effective medications is beneficial for clients, such as Wellbutrin®, which is approved for treating depression and nicotine addiction.

Treatment Centers

Different types of treatment centers are used for SUD, including therapeutic communities, free-standing residential treatment centers, hospital-based rehabilitation units, and long-term residential treatment.

- Hospital-Based Rehabilitation Units: Focus on stabilizing the client in a hospital setting. The average length of stay is 5 to 7 days. Individuals admitted to these units generally have developed medical and psychiatric problems associated with their SUD.
- Therapeutic Communities: Focus on a mental health approach and use broad-based community programs to implement rehabilitation through mutual support, peer pressure and positive role models. This treatment process was initiated in the 1960s, and the implementation of the 12-step program into the

treatment modality was incorporated by AA member Charles E. Dederich. Treatment approaches also include medication and educational groups that embrace mental health issues.

- Free-Standing Residential Treatment Centers: Focus on 24-hour inpatient care. They are stand-alone programs that specialize in the treatment of SUD and dual-diagnosis clients. The clients stay in the facility full time under the supervision of a team of SUD professionals.
- Long-Term Residential Treatment Centers: Focus on long-term treatment for individuals who have completed a residential SUD treatment program and require additional treatment. The average length of stay typically ranges around 90 days, but some centers can provide services for up to a year. Some criteria for long-term treatment include drug-seeking behavior, relapse, or outstanding clinical issues.[62]

To move forward in addressing the global mental healthcare crisis, we need to ensure that adequate availability of services for comorbid diagnosis are available for individuals who are in need of assistance to improve their quality of life. This process will be elaborated on in more depth later in the book.

BOX 4.2 A Critical Thinking Synopsis—Do You Agree?

Again, comorbidity is a global problem, with multifactorial dynamics contributing to a dual diagnosis. As pointed out at the beginning of the chapter, mental illness can lead to SUD and vice versa. The statistics presented in the chapter substantiate that much more work needs to be done; education is key to decreasing statistics; through education, people could better understand the potential adversities of illicit drug utilization.

Effective community-based services, which we will be discussing later, could help decrease the potential for a dual diagnosis. By effectively managing clients with a mental illness or in recovery from mental decline in a community setting, mental health care professionals could contribute to the improvement of quality of life.

Main Points

1. Deinstitutionalization may also contribute to increased illegal drug utilization, as those inflicted with mental disease attempt to self-medicate.
2. The term comorbidity is defined as the presence of two or more diagnoses in a person, which can occur simultaneously or subsequently. In the United States, approximately 9.5 million individuals have both a mental illness and substance use problem.

3. SUD is considered to be a mental illness in and of itself because it alters brain functionality, disrupting an individual's normal hierarchy of needs and desires.
4. Both SUD and mental illness have hereditary factors, making some individuals more susceptible to both during their lifetimes. It has been suggested that genetics, brain neurotransmitter functionality, and environmental factors can contribute to the development of a dual diagnosis.
5. It is believed that only approximately 7.8% of clients attain treatment for both issues. Approximately half of the individuals (51.4%) with a dual diagnosis (comorbidity) do not obtain treatment for either disorder.
6. Scientific research conducted on the treatment of comorbidity reveals that the medical team should treat both diagnoses concurrently. Even when the comorbidities do not occur simultaneously, research demonstrates that psychiatric conditions increase the vulnerability to substance misuse, and substance misuse constitutes a risk factor for subsequent psychiatric illness.

Notes

1. National Institute of Health (2021), *Why is there comorbidity between substance use disorders and mental illness?* https://www.drugabuse.gov/publications/research-reports/common-comorbities-substance-use (accessed November 22, 2021).
2. Patterson, Eric, MSCP, NCC, LPC (2018), *Dual diagnosis substance abuse and mental illness treatment, mental health and drug abuse,* http://www.drugabuse.com/mental-health-drug-abuse (accessed June 5, 2018).
3. Substance Abuse and Mental Health Services Administration (2020), *Key substance use and mental health indicators in the United States: Results from the 2019 national survey on drug use and health* (HHS Publication No. PEP19-5068, NSDUH Series H-54), Center for Behavioral Health Statistics and Quality, http://www.samhsa.gov/data/sites/default/reports/SAMHSA_digital_download/PEP2909709109910PDF.pdf (accessed May 2, 2021), pp. 64.
4. National Center for Drug Abuse Statistics (2019), *Drug abuse statistics,* https://www.drugabusestatistics.org (accessed November 22, 2021).
5. Elflein, John (2023), *Illicit drug use disorder among adults in the United States as of 2021, by level of mental illness,* https://www.statista.com/statistics/252473/us-iilicit-drug-dependence-or-abuse-by-level-of-mental-illness/ (accessed August 20, 2023).
6. Substance Abuse and Mental Health Services Administration (2023), *SAMHSA announces national survey on drug use and health (NSDUH) results detailing mental illness and substance use levels in 2021,* https://www.samhsa.gov/newsroom/press-announcements/20230104/samhsa-announces-nsduh-results-detailing-mental-illness-substance-use-levels-2021 (accessed August 20, 2023).
7. Office for Health Improvement and Disparities (2021), National statistics: Adult substance misuse treatment statistics 2020 to 2021L report, https://www.gov.uk/government/statistics/

substance-misuse-treatment-for-adults-statistics-2020-to-2021/adult-substance-misuse-treatment-statistics-2020-to-2021-report (accessed August 20, 2023).

8. Australian Institute of Health and Welfare (2023), *Alcohol, tobacco, and other drugs in Australia*, https://www.aihw.gov.au/reports/alcohol/alcohol-tobacco-other-drugs-australia/contents/priority-populations/people-with-mental-health-conditions (accessed August 20, 2023).

9. Khan, Saeeda (2017), *Concurrent mental and substance use disorders in Canada, Health Rep*, 28(8), PMID: 2904442, https://www.ncbi.nlm.nih.gov/2904442/ (accessed February 19, 2022).

10. Mood Disorders Society of Canada (2019), *Quick facts: Mental illness and addiction in Canada*, https://mdsc.ca/docs/MDSCQuick_Facts_4th_Edition_EN.pdf (accessed August 20, 2023), pp. 33.

11. Torrens, Marta, et al. (2015), *Comorbidity of substance use and mental disorders in Europe, European Monitoring Centre for Drugs and Drug Addiction*, Luxembourg Publications Office of the European Union, pp. 40.

12. Substance Abuse and Mental Health Services Administration (2016), *Impact of the DSM-IV to DSM-5 changes on the national survey on drug use and health*, https://www.ncbi.nlm.nih.gov/books/NBK519702/ (accessed August 20, 2023).

13. Esper, LH and Furtado, EF (2013), Gender differences and association between psychological stress and alcohol consumption: A systematic review, *J Alcoholism Drug Depend* 1, 116, https://doi.org/10.4172/2329-6488.1000116, pp. 1–5.

14. Peltier, MacKenzie, et al. (2019), Sex differences in stress-related alcohol use, *Neurobiol Stress*, Feb; 10:100149, PMCID: PMC6430711, https://doi.org/10.1016/j.ynstr.2019.100149, https://pubmed,ncbi.nlm.nih.gov/309495621/ (accessed May 5, 2021).

15. Substance Abuse and Mental Health Services Administration (2021), *Key substance use and mental health indicators in the United States: Results from the 2020 national survey on drug use and health*, (HHS Publication No. PEP21-07-01-003, NSDUH Series H-56), Center for Behavioral Health Statistics and Quality, http://www.samhsa.gov/data/sites/default/reports/rpt353191/2020NSDUH FFR1PDFW102121.pdf (accessed May 2, 2021), pp. 1.

16. Ritchie, Hannah and Roser, Max (revised 2022), *Alcohol consumption*, Our World in Data, https://ourworldindata.org/alcohol-consumption (accessed April 26, 2022).

17. Wagner, Steve (2012), *State hospitals are still snake pits of patient abuse, betrayal of the public.* Psychiatric Crime Database, https://www.psychcrime.org/articles/index.php?vd=12 (accessed February 6, 2020).

18. National Institute on Alcohol Abuse and Alcoholism (2022), *Alcohol facts and statistics*, https://www.niaaa.nih.gov/publications/brochures-and-fact-sheets/alcohol-facts-and-statistics (accessed May 2, 2022).

19. National Institute on Alcohol Abuse and Alcohol Addiction (2023), *Alcohols effects on health, global burden*, https://www.niaaa.nih.gov/alcohols-effects-health/alcohol-topics/alcohol-facts-and-statistics/global-burden (accessed August 20, 2023).

20. Elflein, John (2022), *Key facts on alcohol-related deaths worldwide as of 2022*, https://statista.com/ststistics/367890/alcohol-related-deaths-facts-worldwide/ (accessed August 24, 2023).

21. United Nations Office on Drugs and Crimes (2021), *World drug report. Drug market trend: Cannabis, opioids, sales No. E.20.XL.6*, https://www.unodc.org/unodc/en/data-and-analysis/wdr-2021_booklet-3.html (accessed May 2, 2022), pp. 11.
22. World Drug Report (2021), Global Overview of Drug Demand and Drug Supply: United Nations Office on Drugs and Crime, Sales No. E.21.XI.8, https://www.unodc.org/res/wdr2021/field/WDR21_Booklet_2.pdf (accessed May 2, 2022), pp. 22.
23. Pelayo-Terán, José María, et al. (2010), Catechol-O-methyltransferase (COMT) Val158Met variations and cannabis use in first-episode non-affective psychosis: clinical-onset implications, *Psychiatry Res*, 79(3), 291–296, https://pubmed.ncbi.nlm.nih.gov/20493536/#:~:text=The%20Val158Met%20polymorphism%20of%20the%20COMT%20%28Catechol-O-Methyltransferase%29%20gene%2C,use%20in%20the%20modulation%20of%20risk%20of%20psychosis (accessed May 2, 2021).
24. National Institute on Drug Abuse (2021), *Marijuana: Is there a link between marijuana use and psychiatric disorders?* https://www.drugabuse.gov/publications/research-reports/marijuana (accessed May 2, 2021).
25. Zerrin, Atakan (2012), Cannabis, a complex plant: Different compounds and different effects on individuals, *Ther Adv Psychopharmacol*, Dec, 2(6), https://doi.org/10.1177/2045125312457586, https://pubmed.ncbi.nlm.nih.gov/23983983/ (accessed May 20, 2020), pp. 241–254
26. Drug-Free World (2017), *How marijuana has changed over time*, http://www.drugfreeworld.org/course/lesson/th e-truth-about-marijuana/it-s-background/html (accessed June 5, 2020).
27. Cash, Mary, et al. (2020), Mapping cannabis potency in medical and recreational programs in the United States, *PLoSOne*, 2020; 15(3): e0230167, National Center for Biotechnology information, https://ncbi.nlm.nih.gov/32214334 (accessed May 2, 2021).
28. PBS, *Marijuana in the body: A fact sheet on the effects of marijuana*, Partnership for a Drug Free America, https://www.pbs.org/wgbh/pages/frontline/shows/dope/body/effects.html#:~:-text=An%20average%20marijuana%20cigarette%20contains%2030%20nanograms%20of,damaged%20the%20body%20becomes%20more%20susceptible%20to%20cancer (accessed August 20, 2023).
29. PBS, *Marijuana in the body: A fact sheet on the effects of marijuana*, Partnership for a Drug Free America, https://www.pbs.org/wgbh/pages/frontline/shows/dope/body/effects.html#:~:-text=An%20average%20marijuana%20cigarette%20contains%2030%20nanograms%20of,damaged%20the%20body%20becomes%20more%20susceptible%20to%20cancer (accessed August 20, 2023).
30. Center for Disease Control and Prevention (2023), *What we know about marijuana*, https://www.cdc.gov/marijuana/featured-topics/what-we-know-about-marijuana.html (accessed August 20, 2023).
31. American Addiction Centers (2022), *Highest drug use by city*, https://www.addictioncenters.org/blog/substance-abuse-by-city (accessed May 2, 2022).
32. World Drug Report (2021), *Global overview of drug demand and drug supply*, United Nations Office on Drugs and Crime, Sales No. E.21.XI.8, https://www.unodc.org/res/wdr2021/field/WDR21_Booklet_2.pdf (accessed May 2, 2022), pp. 22.

33. Deutsche Welle Organization (2018), *U.S. and Colombia aim to halve cocaine production in five years*, https://www..dw.com/en/us-and-colombia-aim-to-halve-cocaine-production-in-five-years/a-42793844 (accessed May 2, 2021).
34. Addiction Center (2021), *Statistics on addiction in America*, Recovery Worldwide, LLC, https://www.addictioncenter.com/addiction/addiction-statistics/ (accessed May 2, 2021).
35. National Institute on Drug Abuse (2022), *What is the scope of methamphetamine use in the United States?*, https://www.nida.nih.gov/publications/research-reports/methamphetamine (accessed April 22, 2022).
36. Centers for Disease Control and Prevention (2023), *Data: The drug overdose epidemic behind the numbers*, https://www.cdc.gov/opioids/data/index/html (accessed August 20, 2023).
37. National Center for Drug Abuse Statistics (2023), *Opioid epidemic: Addiction statistics*, https://drugabusestatistics.org/opioid-epidemic/ (accessed August 20, 2023).
38. National Center for Drug Abuse Statistics (2023), *Opioid epidemic: Addiction statistics*, https://drugabusestatistics.org/opioid-epidemic/ (accessed August 20, 2023).
39. United Nations Office on Drugs and Crime (2022), *World drug report: Drug market trends cannabis and opioids*, https://reliefweb.int/report/world/unodc-world-drug-report-2022 (accessed August 20, 2023), pp.78
40. Jayawardana, Sahan, et al. (2021), Global consumption of prescription opioid analgesics between 2009–2019: A country-level observational study, *Eclinicalmedicine*, 42, https://doi.org/10.1016/j.eclinm.2021.101198 2589-5370/ (accessed August 20, 2023).
41. World Health Organization (2021), *Opioid overdose*, https://www.who.int/news-room/fact-sheets/detail/opioid-overdose (accessed August 20, 2023).
42. Alliance for Consumer Education (2020), *How prevalent is inhalant abuse in the United States?*, https://www.consumered.org/programs/inhalant-abuse-prevention/data-research# (accessed September 14, 2021).
43. Centers for Disease Control and Prevention (2022), *People with mental health conditions, fact sheet*, United States Department of Health and Human Services, https://www.cdc.gov/tobacco/campaign.tips/groups/people-with-mental-conditions (accessed September 4, 2022).
44. Ding, Jack and Hu, Kevin (2021), *Cigarette smoking and schizophrenia: Etiology, clinical, pharmacological, treatment implications*, 2021, ID: 7698030, https://doi,org/10.1155/2021/769830 (accessed September 5, 2022), pp.1–8.
45. World Population Review (2022), *Smoking rates by country 2022*, https://www.worldpopulationreview.com/country-rankings/smoking-rates-by-country (accessed April 27, 2022).
46. Centers for Disease Control and Prevention (2022), *Smoking and tobacco use, fast facts*, National Center for Chronic Disease Prevention and Health Promotion, https://www.cdc.gov/tobacco/data_statistics/fact_sheets/fast_facts/index.html (accessed August 19, 2022).
47. Center for integrated Health Care (2013), *Hallucinogens–LSD, peyote, psilocybin, and PCP*, https://www.mirecc.va.gov/cih-visn2/Documents/Provider_Education_Handouts/Hallucinogens_Information_Sheet_for_BHPs_Version_3.pdf (accessed May 2, 2021),
48. Substance Abuse and Mental Health Services Administration (2021), *Key substance use and mental health indicators in the United States: Results from the 2020 national survey on drug*

use and health (HHS Publication No. PEP21-07-01-003, NSDUH Series H-56), Center for Behavioral Health Statistics and Quality, http://www.samhsa.gov/data/sites/default/reports/rpt353191/2020NSDUHFFR1PDFW102121.pdf (accessed May 2, 2021), pp. 2.

49. Substance Abuse and Mental Health Services Administration (2021 *Key substance use and mental health indicators in the United States: Results from the 2020 national survey on drug use and health*), (HHS Publication No. PEP21-07-01-003, NSDUH Series H-56), Center for Behavioral Health Statistics and Quality, http://www.samhsa.gov/data/sites/default/reports/rpt353191/2020NSDUHFFR1PD FW102121.pdf (accessed May 2, 2021), pp. 2.
50. National Institute on Drug Abuse (2023), *Marijuana and hallucinogen use, binge drinking reach historic highs among adults 30 to 50,* https://nida.nih.gov/news-events/news-releases/2023/08/marijuana-and-hallucinogen-use-binge-drinking-reached-historic-highs-among-adults-35-to-50 (accessed August 20, 2023).
51. National Institute on Drug Abuse (2023), *Marijuana and hallucinogen use, binge drinking reach historic highs among adults 30 to 50,* https://nida.nih.gov/news-events/news-releases/2023/08/marijuana-and-hallucinogen-use-binge-drinking-reached-historic-highs-among-adults-35-to-50 (accessed August 20, 2023).
52. Lukacovic, Marek and Masaryk, Radomir (2021), Use of hallucinogens in Slovakia: Does it differ from global trends?, *International Journal of Drug Policy,*98, https://doi.org/10.1016/j.drugpo.2021.103385 (accessed August 20, 2023).
53. National Institute on Drug Abuse (2010), *Comorbidity: Addiction and other mental illness, research reports,* https://drugabuse.gov /publications/research-reports/comorbidity-addiction-other-mental-illness (accessed August 22, 2018).
54. National Institute on Drug Abuse (2010), *Comorbidity: Addiction and other mental illness, research reports,* https://drugabuse.gov/publications/research-reports/comorbidity-addiction-other-mental-illness (accessed August 22, 2018).
55. National Institute on Drug Abuse (2010), *Comorbidity: Addiction and other mental illness, research reports,* https://drugabuse.gov/publications/research-reports/comorbidity-addiction-other-mental-illness (accessed August 22, 2018).
56. National Institute on Drug Abuse (2010), *Comorbidity: Addiction and other mental illness, research reports,* https://drugabuse.gov/publications/research-reports/comorbidity-addiction-other-mental-illness (accessed August 22, 2018).
57. National Center for Drug Abuse Statistics (2022), *Drug use among youth: Facts and statistics,* https://www.drugabusestatistics.org/teen-drug-use (accessed April 22, 2022).
58. Substance Abuse and Mental Health Services Administration (2021), *Key substance use and mental health indicators in the United States: Results from the 2020 national survey on drug use and health* (HHS Publication No. PEP21-07-01-003, NSDUH Series H-56), Center for Behavioral Health Statistics and Quality, http://www.samhsa.gov/data/sites/default/reports/rpt353191/2020NS DUHFFR1PDFW102121.pdf (accessed May 2, 2021), pp. 3.
59. Substance Abuse and Mental Health Services Administration (2020), *Key substance use and mental health indicators in the United States: Results from the 2019 national survey on drug use and health* (HHS Publication No. PEP19-5068, NSDUH Series H-54), Center for Behavioral Health Statistics and Quality, http://www.samhsa.gov/data/sites/default/reports/SAMHSA_digital_download/PEP2909709109910PDF.pdf (accessed May 2, 2021), pp. 65.

60. Joint Commission on Administrative rules, Administrative Code. Title 77, Public Health, Part 2060: Alcoholism and substance abuse treatment and intervention licenses, Section 2060.401, levels of care, Section 2060.201.142. https://www.ilga.gov/commission/jcar/admincode/077/07702060sections.html (accessed October 19, 2021).

61. National Institute on Drug Abuse (2021), *What are the treatments for comorbid substance use disorder and mental health conditions?* https://www.nidanih.gov/publications/research-reports/common-comorbidities-substance-use-disorders/what-are-the-treatments-for-comorbid-substance-use (accessed October 19, 2021).

62. Recovery Connection (2011), *Addiction treatment modalities and programs*, https://www.recoveryconnection.com/addiction-treatment-modalities/ (accessed October 19, 2021).

Credits

Fig. 4.1: Data Source: https://ourworldindata.org/alcohol-consumption.
Fig. 4.2: Data Source: https://www.unodc.org/res/wdr2021/field/WDR21_Booklet_2.pdf.
Fig. 4.3: Data Source: https://www.unodc.org/res/wdr2021/field/WDR21_Booklet_2.pdf.
Fig. 4.4: Source: https://reliefweb.int/report/world/unodc-world-drug-report-2022.
Fig. 4.5: Data Source: https://www.worldpopulationreview.com/country-rankings/smoking-rates-by-country.

CHAPTER 5

COVID-19 and Mental Health

The main objective of this chapter is for the reader to understand how life circumstances and viruses can impact mental health and how pandemics can alter the delivery of mental health services.

The COVID-19 pandemic exacerbated the mental healthcare crisis worldwide; information in this chapter reveals how pandemics and social consequences can impact mental health, why mental health screening processes are important, and how pandemics influence the delivery of mental healthcare services.

Globally, there was an increase in individuals experiencing mental health decline because of isolative practices implemented with the pandemic, employment loss, decreased income, and intensity of stress. A global study encompassing 204 countries revealed that in 2020, there were 76.2 million additional anxiety conditions and 53.2 million additional major depressive illnesses diagnosed.[1]

It was reported by WHO that people with preexisting mental conditions were more likely to be hospitalized because of COVID-19 and have a severe viral illness episode, especially if there was a psychosis or bipolar illness diagnosis. It was recommended in 2020 that these individuals needed to be viewed as high risk for a terminal infection process. People with mental conditions many times have comorbidities, and this dynamic may increase the severity of the symptomatology of the COVID-19 virus.

United States Impact

As of January 2024, the COVID-19 pandemic had resulted in 110 million positive cases and over 1 million deaths in America.[2] The COVID-19 pandemic is being considered the worst pandemic in U.S. history, exceeding the death toll (675,000 Americans) of the 1918 Spanish flu. There was also a 7-day average of 52,293 positive COVID test results out of 556,305 tests performed in May of 2022, and the number of people hospitalized because of COVID was 15,999, with 1,801 in intensive care units.[3] Impacts on mental well-being have been noted in adults, children, and adolescents, with various reasons noted for the decline in mental wellness.

Adults

A Kaiser Family Foundation Health Tracking Poll from July of 2020 found that many adults were experiencing negative impacts on their mental health and well-being. These included 36% reported having difficulty with sleeping, decreased food consumption was noted in 32% of the individuals surveyed, increased alcohol consumption or substance use was noted in 12% of individuals, and 12% of people experienced worsening of chronic conditions.[4] Figure 5.1 illustrates the percentages of mental health deterioration by gender during COVID-19.

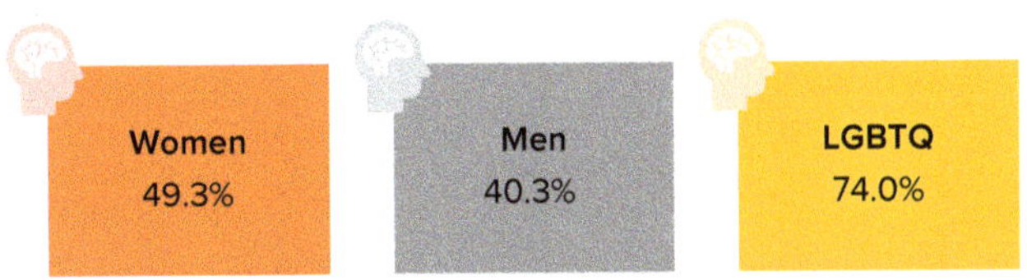

FIGURE 5.1 U.S. Reported Gender Mental Health Deterioration During COVID-19 Pandemic[5,6]

In January of 2021, 41% of adults reported symptoms of anxiety and/or a depressive condition.[7] Then, in March of 2022, a new survey showed some decline in negative mental health adversities, with only 31.9% of adults reporting symptoms of an anxiety or depressive condition.[8] Most data and reporting of statistics confirmed that women's mental health was being impacted significantly more than men's. Some individuals are attributing this dynamic to the rise in domestic violence statistics and to the increase in familial environmental stress related to school closures.

Suicidal Ideation

Suicidal thoughts or ideas that encompassed individuals contemplating, wishing, or being preoccupied with death increased during the pandemic. Suicidal thoughts are a risk factor for planning a suicide and should be taken seriously. During 2021, 11% of adults reported experiencing suicidal ideation.[9] America has one of the highest suicide rates among wealthy countries. The CDC reported in 2021 that the total number of suicides in the United States during 2020 was 45,855.[10] President Joe Biden declared September 10th, 2021, "World Suicide Prevention Day" to call upon Americans to take action to prevent suicide. Figure 5.2 illustrates the suicide rates in the United States.

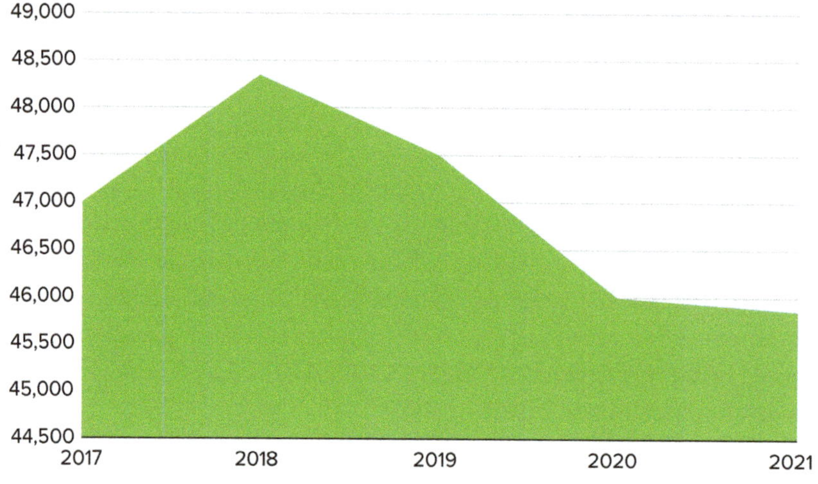

FIGURE 5.2 Suicide Rates in the United States[11, 12, 13]

Self-Harming Behaviors

Self-harming behaviors are used by individuals sometimes when they are attempting to handle difficult feelings, experiencing psychological pain, or are overwhelmed. Some people explain that self-harming provides a temporary release to a current problem or feeling. Examples of self-harming behaviors include cutting, scratching, burning, carving, self-hitting, head banging, piercing skin, and inserting objects under the skin. It is estimated that approximately 5% of the adult population performs self-harming behaviors.[14] Self-harming behaviors can exist on a spectrum from no suicide intent to high levels of intent; thus, they must be viewed seriously. The increase in self-harming behaviors during COVID-19 could be attributed to increased stress and multiple losses.

Increased Substance Misuse

A June 2020 survey revealed that 13% of adults experienced new or increased substance use related to the pandemic.[15] In 2022, it is believed that the percentage increased to 29% in America. Those individuals with a substance use disorder diagnosis prior to the pandemic were at a higher risk of adverse consequences. A provisional statistic reported by the CDC revealed that there were an estimated 107,622 drug overdose deaths in 2021, an increase of 15% from 2020 (93,655).[16] An increase is also noted from the previous year; overdose deaths in 2019 were 70,630.[17] It is believed that the majority of the overdoses were related to synthetic opioids (fentanyl). There were also increases in the utilization of alcohol, heroin, methamphetamines, and cocaine during the pandemic. An illustration of drug overdose deaths in the United States is provided in Figure 5.3.

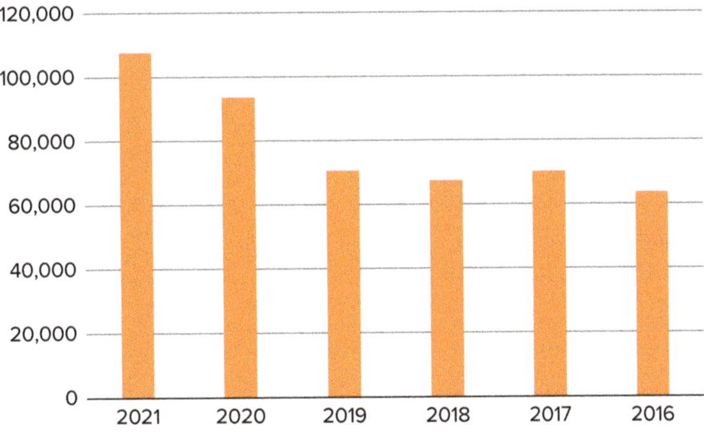

FIGURE 5.3 Drug Overdose Deaths United States[18, 19]

Children and Adolescents

Children and Adolescents are more likely to experience anxiety and depression during and after a pandemic. In 2020, it was reported by the CDC that mental health-related emergency room visits increased 24% from 2019 for children 5 to 11 years of age and 31% for those ages 12 to 17 years old.[20] A Kaiser Family Foundation study concluded that during the pandemic, 25% of high school students reported worsened emotional and cognitive health, and more than 20% of parents with children 5 to 12 years of age reported their children experienced worsened mental or emotional health.[21]

New data released by the CDC revealed in 2021 that more than a third (37%) of high school students reported they experienced poor mental health during the COVID-19 pandemic, and 44% reported they persistently felt sad or hopeless during the past year.[22]

The American Academy of Pediatrics, the American Academy of Child and Adolescent Psychiatry, and the Children's Hospital Association have joined together to declare a National State of Emergency in Children's Mental Health. The agencies identified issues such as federal funding, telehealth, school-based mental health care, integrated mental health care with primary care pediatrics, reducing the risk of suicide, trauma-informed care, workforce challenges, and policies.[23]

It is also reported that the number of child suicide attempts and self-injury cases increased in the first three quarters of 2021; the rate was 47% higher among children 5 to 8 years of age and 182% higher among 9- to 12-year-olds.[24] Out of the 44.2% of high school students who experienced persistent feelings of sadness or hopelessness in 2021, almost 20% seriously considered suicide, and 9% attempted suicide during the pandemic.[25] A study published in the *Journal of the American Medical Association of Pediatrics* stated, "Georgia, Indiana, New Jersey, Oklahoma, and Virginia had an increase in absolute count of adolescent suicides during the pandemic. These states, along with California, also had an increase in the proportion of overall suicide attempts among adolescents."[26]

Substance misuse is an ongoing issue with children and adolescents without a pandemic. A research team in California conducting an ABCD study on youth and substance misuse revealed that adolescent alcohol utilization declined during the pandemic, but nicotine and prescription drug utilization increased.[27] Another study, based on 49 published sources, concluded that the overall prevalence of youth alcohol, cannabis, tobacco, and e-cigarette/vaping use declined during the pandemic.[28] The researchers believe that a more in-depth analysis of the decrease in substance misuse needs to be evaluated with regard to peer influences and parental supervision.

The long-term effects on children's mental well-being from the COVID-19 pandemic are yet to be seen, but the longevity of experienced trauma associated with isolative practices has already demonstrated concerning statistics. Compounding the isolative problem with potential ACEs, such as domestic abuse, substance misuse caretakers, and being quarantined with family members that experience mental illness, there is the potential for additional negative impacts for children as they progress into adulthood.

Global Impact

The worldwide impact of COVID-19 will be observed for years after the pandemic is resolved. Globally, COVID-19 (2024) has resulted in 702 million positive cases and nearly 7 million deaths.[29] On May 8th, 2022, there were approximately 259 thousand new cases of COVID-19 worldwide.[30] Statista reported that as of September 12th, 2022 the number of COVID-19 tests that had been performed globally are massive: United Kingdom: 522,526,476; France: 271,490,188; Germany 122,332,384; USA: 1,108,655,515; Italy: 243,962,017; Russia: 273,400,000; Spain: 471,036,328; and China: 160,000,000.[31] The emergence of different variants of the COVID-19 virus sustains ongoing adversities in all countries.

Adults

An International Committee of the Red Cross Survey revealed that 51% of the respondents in Colombia, Lebanon, the Philippines, South Africa, Switzerland, Ukraine, and the United Kingdom reported that the COVID-19 pandemic had impacted their mental health.[32] WHO estimated in 2020 that worldwide, the COVID-19 pandemic had resulted in a 27.6% increase in major depressive conditions and a 25.6% increase in anxiety conditions being diagnosed.[33]

A 2021 worldwide analysis published in *Scientific Reports* estimated the global prevalence of depression at 28%, 26.9% for anxiety, 24.1% for post-traumatic stress symptoms, 36.5% for stress, 50% for psychological distress, and 27.6% for sleep problems.[34] As in the United States, there were noted gender differences related to mental well-being in Spain; several studies have found that compared to men, women presented higher emotional discomfort, worse mental health status, worse psychological responses to the pandemic, and higher emotional vulnerability to the effects of the lockdown period.[35]

Suicidal Ideation

Globally, approximately one million people die from suicide every year. A study in Australia revealed that thoughts of suicide occurred in 18% of the population across the acute phase of the pandemic and decreased to 16.2% in 2021.[36] Another study in Canada, England, Belgium, Switzerland, Hong Kong, the Philippines, New Zealand and the United States on suicidal ideation reported that 14.7% of individuals had thoughts of being better off dead or harming themselves on several days, 6.4% over half the days, and 3.6% nearly every day.[37] Five months later, the same study illustrated an increase in suicidal ideation, with 15.3% having self-harming thoughts on several days, 7.8% on over half the days, and 4.4% nearly every day.[38] Figure 5.4 depicts the countries with the highest suicide rates.

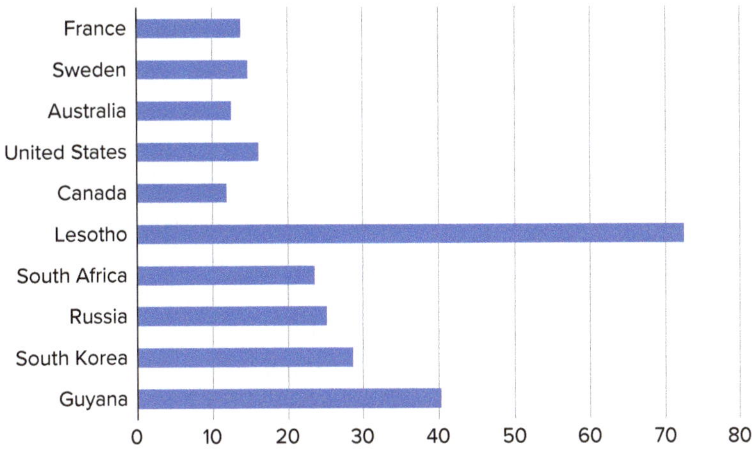

FIGURE 5.4 Global Suicide Rates per Country[39]

In 2021, 1,295 men and 564 women died of suicide in the Netherlands; this was an average of 5 suicides per day.[40] In Northern Ireland, there was a 33.6% increase in suicides from 2019 to 2020.[41]

Self-Harming Behaviors

There has also been an increase in self-harming behaviors globally. The United Kingdom had an increase in thoughts of self-harming behaviors, with 26.1% of 18- to 29-year-old adults reporting experiencing thoughts of wanting to hurt themselves and 7.9% of adults 45 to 59 years of age.[42] In Nepal, emergency room visits for self-harming behaviors increased by 71.9% in 2020 from March to June.[43] It has been identified in numerous studies that loneliness, coping patterns, preexisting mental health conditions, demographics, and employment status were all adversities predictive of self-harming behaviors. Four in ten Indonesians reported having thoughts of self-harm related to loneliness during the pandemic.[44] A few studies, such as one in

Lebanon, had no identified results of increased self-harming behaviors among the individuals in their research.

Increased Substance Misuse

The 2021 *World Drug Report* revealed that the COVID-19 pandemic led to shifts in drug utilization overall; MDMA (Ecstasy), LSD, and cocaine utilization decreased because of the closure of social and recreational venues, cannabis use increased, an increase in nonmedical and pharmaceutical drug use was noted, and alcohol consumption increased. It was also noted in the 2020 study that there was a 64% increase in the use of pharmaceutical sedatives in the surveyed countries, while cocaine use decreased in 30% of the countries.[45]

A study of older adults (50–59 years old) in Ghana revealed that 16% of the adults initiated or increased their consumption of alcohol or tobacco during the COVID-19 pandemic.[46] An initiated or increased use of cannabis, cigarettes, and e-cigarettes among younger adults living alone during COVID was also noted in Canada.[47]

Again, worldwide, about 0.5 million deaths annually are attributed to drug use, with more than 30% being related to overdose.[48] Increases in drug overdose deaths during the pandemic were noted in Canada (62% were opioid related), the United States, Finland, and Spain.[49] In Canada, drug overdose-related deaths increased by 107% in Alberta, 80% in British Columbia, and 28% in Quebec.[50] Also, there were 1,339 Scotland drug-related deaths in 2020, the largest number ever recorded.[51] Figure 5.5 illustrates some countries that had an increase in overdose deaths in 2020.

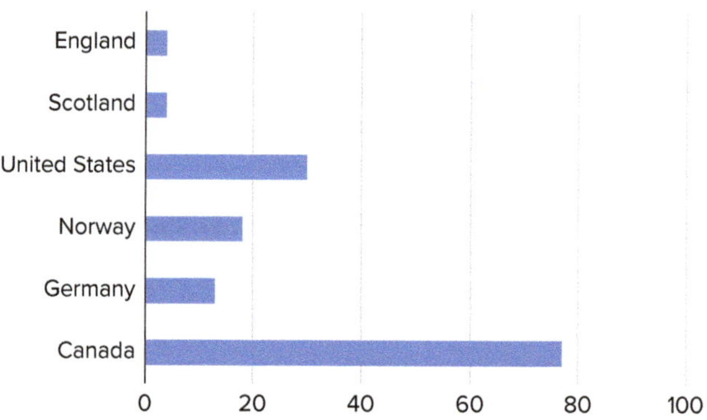

FIGURE 5.5 Increase in Overdose Deaths 2020[52]

Children and Adolescents

Worldwide, the impact of COVID-19 on the mental health of children and adolescents has been profound. More than 16 billion children have suffered some loss of education, with at least 463 million unable to access remote learning.[53] UNICEF conducted a survey on the mental health impact of adolescents and young people in

Latin America and the Caribbean, with 27% reporting anxiety and 15% reporting depression, with 30% stating the reason base for the emotion being economically related.[54] In Sweden, there is also documentation of higher rates of insomnia and symptoms of depression, anxiety, and eating disorders in adolescents during the COVID-19 pandemic.

A meta-analysis of 16 studies, including East Asia (55.2%), four from Europe (13.8%), six from North America (20.7%), two from Central America and South America (6.9%), and one study from the Middle East (3.4%) revealed clinically elevated depression and anxiety symptoms among children aged 4 to 17 years old at 25.2% and 20.5%, respectively.[55] Figure 5.6 depicts losses incurred by children because of the COVID-19 pandemic.

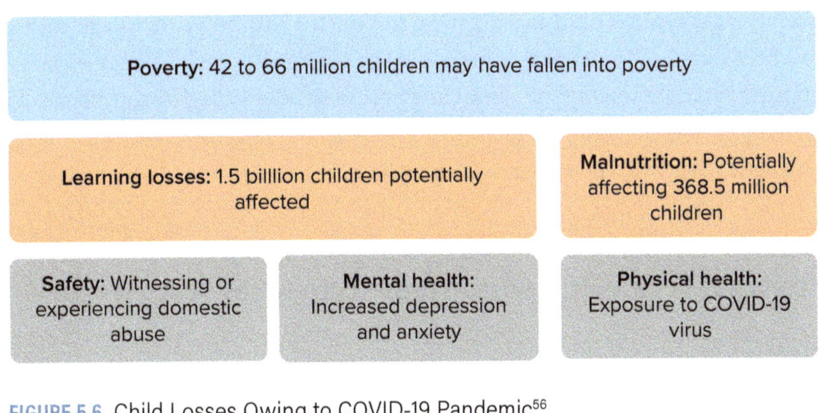

FIGURE 5.6 Child Losses Owing to COVID-19 Pandemic[56]

Research with students in China concluded that the psychological stress response (PSR) was correlated with nonsuicidal self-injury (NSSI) and causing or worsening sleep disorders. This study revealed that 17.6% of the students were experiencing PSR, and 24.9% were experiencing NSSI during the earlier periods of the pandemic.[57] An Australian study revealed that there was a significant increase in children and adolescent admissions to intensive care units with deliberate self-harm in early 2020.[58] In Taiwan, adolescents exhibited a prevalence rate of 40.9% for NSSI.[59] The NSSI rates of Swedish students increased during the collection of data with each subsequent sample obtained I to III; (24.4%) to 2020 (27%) to the spring of 2021 (30.6%).[60]

Worldwide, suicide is the fifth most prevalent cause of death for adolescents aged 10 to 19 years old, resulting in approximately 45,800 deaths annually.[61] A study in England concluded that suicide rates involving children were higher during the first pandemic lockdown period.[62] A CBC news article for Canada reported that McMaster Children's Hospital admissions for medical support after a suicide attempt tripled over a 4-month period during the pandemic.[63] Suicide attempts for adolescents based on emergency department data increased in South Korea from 50.6% to 52.4% for poisoning and 31.2% to 40.5% for cutting.[64] Croatia saw a 57.1% increase in suicides during COVID for the age group 15 to 25 years of age.[65] A pediatric hospital, Bambino Gesu in Rome, noted that the number of hospitalizations for suicide attempts doubled between the 15- to 24-year-old age group during the pandemic.[66]

Globally, substance misuse among youth and adolescents increased in most countries during the COVID pandemic. A Canadian study on substance misuse among youth 16 to 24 years of age concluded that 40% of the sampled youth who use alcohol, cannabis, or both reported increased utilization.[67] The increased utilization of substances was noted in some Indonesian youth, with 53.4% reporting increased alcohol consumption, 17.8% reported increased cigarette smoking, and 30.8% reported increased illicit drug utilization.[68] A southern African country (Zimbabwe) reported that there was an upward trend of drug/substance use among adolescents and youth, including Broncleer® (containing codeine) and methamphetamine.[69] In Italy, the frequency of severe alcohol intoxication in youth 13 to 24 years of age increased from 0.88% during the last part of lockdown to 11.3% after lockdown release. When comparing this data during the same time period in 2019, a highly significant difference emerged, with severe alcohol intoxications accounting for 11.31% of emergency department visits in 2020 versus 2.96% in 2019.[70]

COVID-19 Virus Infection: Mental Health Impacts

In an article by Columbia University, Maura Boldrini, MD, PhD, discusses how the viral infection itself can impact mental health, stating, "I have seen COVID-19 patients with new onset delusions, hallucinations, anxiety, and depression. We think that biological changes like inflammation are linked to our behavior, providing another explanation of how infectious diseases can affect mental health. The body's immune response triggers the release of cytokines that disrupt the production of neurotransmitters and how neurons communicate in the brain. We could be dealing with a mental health pandemic long after the COVID-19 pandemic is over."[71]

Katlyn Nemani, a New York University neuropsychiatrist, states, "It seems like having COVID puts you at higher risk for psychiatric illness after the infection." A study of 69 million individual health records revealed the incidence of any psychiatric diagnosis in the 14 to 90 days after a COVID diagnosis was 18.1%, including 5.8% that was a first-time diagnosis.[72] Some experts believe this might be linked to the peculiarities of COVID-19 and how it can infect the nervous system tissues; others think that viral infections simply can impact mental well-being, and some believe it might be the psychological stress associated with illness.

But we do know that SARS-CoV-2 invades the central nervous system and spreads to the brain and neurons, generating neurodegenerative dysfunctions. While experts still need to further study the effects of COVID-19 on the brain, it has been reported that those with more severe viral symptoms (neuroinflammation, cognitive impairment, loss of smell, and brain stroke) are at a higher risk for post-traumatic stress disorder, anxiety, insomnia, and obsessive-compulsive symptoms.

COVID-19 Mental Health Treatment Adversities Worldwide

Globally, it is reported that there were increased issues related to treatment gaps because of the lack of pandemic preparedness in mental health systems; according to a survey conducted by the World Health Organization, the COVID-19 pandemic had disrupted or halted mental health services in 93% of countries worldwide.[73] The disruptions were widespread in the 130 countries assessed by WHO: 60% reported decreased accessibility to mental health services for vulnerable people, 67% saw disruptions in counseling and psychotherapy, there was a 35% occurrence with adversities in emergency interventions, and accessibility to medications was identified as a problem for 30% of the countries surveyed.[74]

United States

In the United States, there was a decline in the utilization of mental health services in 2020. There was a 34% (14 million children) decline in services used by children under the age of 19 and a 22% (12 million adults) decline in the visits by adults aged 19 to 64.[75] The American federal government expanded access to telehealth, including telemental health, for individuals covered by Medicare and Medicaid programs at the beginning of the COVID-19 pandemic through the end of the public health emergency declaration.

Implementing e-mental health plays an important role in developing efficient health systems that sustain pandemic conditions. President Biden, in his State of the Union address, identified behavioral health adversities and described proposals to strengthen entry and treatment, expand community services, strengthen the workforce, address youth mental health, integrate mental health into primary care, expand access to crisis services, and avoid legal involvement.[76]

Spain

The ability to deliver mental health support in Spain was affected by the pandemic directly and indirectly. Overburdening of health systems led to moving staff from mental health services to COVID-focused tasks. Public health restrictions led to temporary restrictions and restarts in the provision of face-to-face services. And, school closures decreased mental health provisions by limiting staff to provide those services.[77]

Italy

Most of the existing psychiatric wards in hospitals were converted to COVID units in Italy. In 2020, they closed second- and third-level outpatient units (perinatal depression, eating disorders, geriatric psych, adult neuropsychiatry, adult autism), using phone calls and video conferences for emergencies and specific patient requests. General psychiatry outpatient visits were restricted to urgent visits and patients who required medications. In Italy, the psychiatric wards in hospitals that remained open followed all infection control protocols.[78]

Germany

A survey conducted on mental health services in Germany revealed an 80% reduction in inpatient treatment, a 50% reduction in day hospital treatment during the first phase, and a 70% reduction in the second phase of the pandemic. Individual psychotherapy cases decreased by 23% in March of 2020; treatment cases decreased by 30% and group therapy by 60% by April of 2020. Video consultation services were used by 3% of the surveyed facilities before the pandemic, 55% of the facilities introduced them during the pandemic, and 37% planned to continue using them after the pandemic.[79]

China

The National Health Commission in China published several guidelines initiating principles for emergency psychological crisis intervention during the COVID-19 pandemic and then established psychological assistance hotlines. Plus, online mental health services (surveys, counseling, education) were implemented for those in need in China.[80] Another study revealed overall, 63% of mental health service users received services via the internet or telephone, and 83% of participants with perceived mental health needs ascribed their lack of help-seeking to barriers in accessibility and availability.[81]

Mental Health Screening

It has been recommended that voluntary screening for mental health decline should be implemented in primary care practice, as well as in general hospitals, because of the impact of COVID-19. The screening should be used with children, adolescents, and adults. For children, there is the Depression Scale for Children that screens for depression in ages 6 to 17 years; the Pediatric Symptom Check to identify cognitive, emotional, and behavioral problems in children 4 to 16 years of age; the Spence Children's Anxiety Scale that screens for six kinds of anxiety in school-age and preschool children; and the CRAFFT behavioral health screening tool that screens for high-risk alcohol and other drug use disorders in children and adolescents.

For adults, there is the Depression Screening Tool, Generalized Anxiety Disorder-7, Substance Abuse Screening, and the Mental Health Screening Form III. If the screening reveals a low to moderate impact on mental well-being, referrals to community mental health providers should be implemented. Identification of any crisis situation should be referred for potential inpatient treatment.

The CDC, National Center for Health Statistics, and the Census Bureau implemented the "Household Pulse Survey" in April of 2020 to gather data on the mental health impact of COVID-19. In October of 2020, symptoms of anxiety or depression were reported in 41.8% of females and 30.3% of males. In January of 2021, the data revealed symptoms in 39.5% of females and 32.4% of males. April of 2021 exposed that 31% of females and 23% of males still experienced symptoms of anxiety and/or depression. And in April of 2022, symptoms of depression and anxiety were still reported by 30.4% of females and 22.8% of males.[82]

Mental Health America created an online screening program in 2014. In 2020, over 2.6 million people took the mental health screen, comprising the largest dataset compiled for a mental health help-seeking population during the pandemic. And, representing a nearly 200% increase over the number of people who completed a screening in 2019. Out of the individuals who screened positive for depression or anxiety, only 36% reported seeking treatment.[83] It was also identified that loneliness and isolation (71% of screens), past trauma (53% of screens), and relationship problems (42% of screens) were the top three concerns related to their mental health concerns.[84]

COVID-19 Impact on Healthcare Providers

A study by the Kaiser Family Foundation revealed that 93% of healthcare workers were experiencing stress, 86% anxiety, 77% frustration, 78% exhaustion and burnout, and 76% felt overwhelmed.[85] Other studies conducted in the United States regarding healthcare workers revealed similar results. The Lorna Breen Health Care Provider Protection Act was signed into law on March 18th, 2022, for resources to reduce and prevent healthcare professional suicides, burnout, and behavioral health disorders. Figure 5.7 illustrates the number of healthcare workers infected with COVID-19 by May 8th, 2020.

A Chinese healthcare worker study reported high rates of depression (50%), anxiety (45%), insomnia (34%) and distress (72%).[87] Studies from Italy and France reported a high prevalence of depressive symptoms, post-traumatic stress disorder, and burnout.[88] Healthcare workers in Iraq, Egypt, Somalia, Sudan, Yemen, Jordan, Pakistan, Afghanistan, and Morocco exhibited symptoms of depression (57.5%), stress (42%), and anxiety (59.1%).[89] In Wuhan, China, there was a 75.3% overall prevalence of psychiatric manifestations (anxiety, depression, sleep disturbances) in a population of healthcare workers employed in a tertiary hospital during the SARS-CoV-2 outbreak.[90]

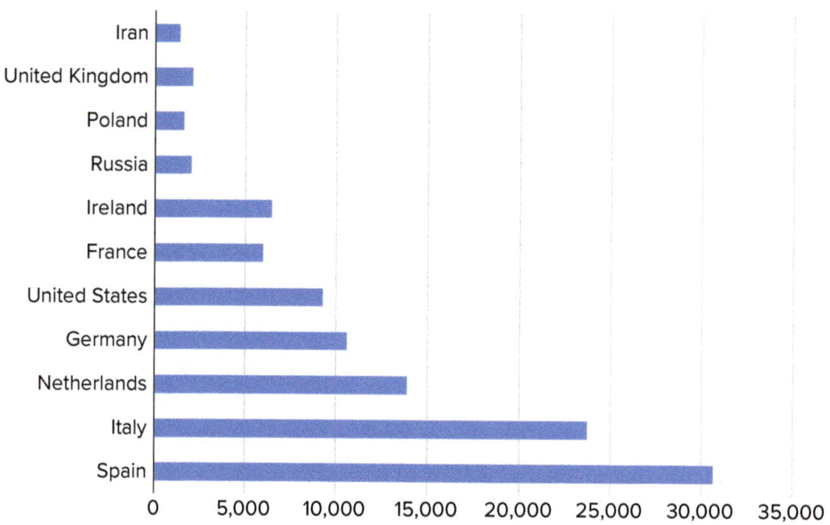

FIGURE 5.7 Number of Healthcare Workers Infected with COVID-19[86]

The European Commission released an opinion on supporting the mental health of healthcare workers in 2021, *Supporting Mental Health of Health Workforce and Other Essential Workers: Opinion of the Expert Panel on Effective Ways of Investing in Health,* that offers advice and interventions for maintaining healthcare worker mental well-being. Figure 5.8 depicts the number of healthcare worker deaths from COVID-19 by May 7th, 2020.

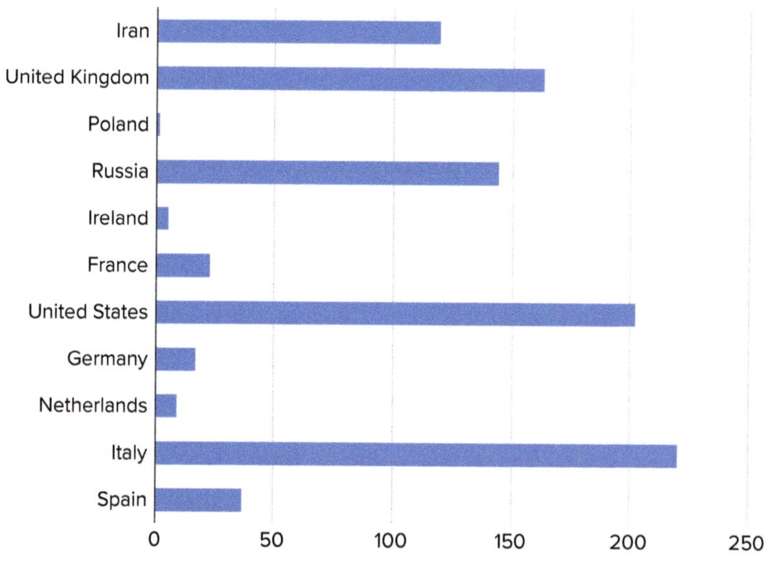

FIGURE 5.8 Healthcare Worker Deaths by May 7th, 2020[91]

Pandemics: Long-Term Consequences

History has provided evidence that there are long-lasting consequences of pandemics. Plus, illogical decision-making and poor leadership in countries could multiply the harmful effects of COVID-19. The Black Plague, which occurred in the 14th century, resulted in a massive decline in population because of the number of deaths and changes in social, economic, and religious structures. It is estimated that between one third and one half of the European population (25 million) died from that outbreak.

The Spanish flu that occurred between 1918 and 1920 claimed an estimated 40 million lives worldwide, affecting population structure and economics. With regard to the economic impact, it is suggested that the real per capita gross domestic product was reduced by 6% and private consumption by 8%, which led to declines in real returns on stocks globally.

Pandemics cause both short-term and long-term economic impacts in countries, manifesting shocks to economic growth. It has been previously established that the severity of the pandemic does directly correlate with the severity of economic outcomes. Employment loss, economic hardships, and poverty have also been associated with a long-lasting decline in mental health. Long-term complications from the COVID-19 pandemic will most likely impact the mental health of individuals globally for decades.

Steven Taylor, author of *The Psychology of Pandemics: Preparing for the Next Global Outbreak of Infectious Disease* and professor of psychiatry at the University of British Columbia, states, "For an unfortunate minority of people, perhaps 10% to 15%, life will not return to normal, due to the impact of the pandemic on their mental well-being."[92] It is also believed that those suffering from long COVID can experience poor cardiovascular functioning, wide-range neurological symptoms, and chronic fatigue with or without damage to the heart, kidneys, lungs, and brain. Mitigation was more developed for the COVID-19 pandemic versus previous pandemics in the world, so detriments could be fewer. But the global long-term impacts of COVID-19 on mental health and well-being, employment, economy, government, and societal structure are yet to be seen.

BOX 5.1 A Critical Thinking Synopsis—Do You Agree?

The COVID-19 pandemic exacerbated mental health adversities worldwide, resulting in additional strains on the delivery of mental health care services. No country was prepared to handle a pandemic's mental health impact on their populace, which resulted in additional consequences for mental health care recipients.

During this pandemic, all countries increased technology utilization for health care in an attempt to mitigate the public's mental health care needs. So, technology systems have been and are continuing to be strategized as

(continued)

an alternative source to treat clients, which will be discussed in greater detail later in the book.

As far as prevention strategies to deter mental health decline of its populace in countries for future pandemics, there needs to be some type of income system strategized for families that are no longer allowed to work their jobs, improvement in technological educational systems for children, and evaluation of strict isolative protocols for extended periods of time.

Main Points

1. The COVID-19 pandemic exacerbated the mental healthcare crisis. Globally, there was an increase of individuals experiencing an impact on their mental health because of isolative practices implemented with the pandemic, employment loss, decreased income, and intensity of stress.
2. In January of 2021, 41% of American adults reported symptoms of anxiety and/or a depressive condition, and 11% of adults reported experiencing suicidal ideation.
3. In 2020, it was reported by the CDC that mental health-related emergency room visits increased 24% from 2019 for children 5 to 11 years of age and 31% for those ages 12 to 17 years old.
4. A 2021 worldwide analysis published in *Scientific Reports* estimated the global prevalence of depression at 28%, 26.9% for anxiety, 24.1% for post-traumatic stress symptoms, 36.5% for stress, 50% for psychological distress, and 27.6% for sleep problems.
5. The 2021 *World Drug Report* revealed that the COVID-19 pandemic led to shifts in drug utilization overall; MDMA (Ecstasy), LSD, and cocaine utilization decreased because of the closure of social and recreational venues, cannabis use increased, an increase in nonmedical and pharmaceutical drug use was noted, and alcohol consumption increased.
6. Worldwide, the impact of COVID-19 on the mental health of children and adolescents has been profound.
7. Worldwide, substance misuse among youth and adolescents increased in most countries during the COVID pandemic.
8. According to a survey conducted by WHO, the COVID-19 pandemic disrupted or halted mental health services in 93% of countries worldwide.
9. It has been recommended that voluntary screening for mental health decline should be implemented in primary care practice, as well as in general hospitals, because of the impact of COVID-19.

Notes

1. The Lancet (2021), *How the COVID-19 pandemic has affected depression and anxiety around the world*, https://www.thelancet.com/infographics/covid-mental-health (accessed November 30, 2021).
2. Worldometer (2024), *COVID-19 data*, https://www.worldometers.info/coronovirus (accessed January 21, 2024).
3. Ritchie, Hannah, et al. (2022), *Coronavirus disease United States*, https://www.ourworldindata.org/coronavirus. country/united-states (accessed May 14, 2022).
4. Panchal, Nirmita, et al. (2021), *The implications of COVID-19 for mental health and substance use*, Kaiser Family Foundation, https://www.kff.org/coronavirus-covid-19/issue-brief/the-implications-of-covid-19-for-mental-health-and-substance-use/ (accessed November 30, 2021).
5. Panchal, Nirmita, et al. (2021), *The implications of COVID-19 for mental health and substance use*, Kaiser Family Foundation, https://www.kff.org/coronavirus-covid-19/issue-brief/the-implications-of-covid-19-for-mental-health-and-substance-use/ (accessed November 30, 2021).
6. Dawson, Lindsey, et al. (2021), *The impact of the COVID-19 pandemic in LGBT + people's mental health*, Kaiser Family Foundation, https://www/kff.org/other/issue-brief/the-impact-of-the-covid-19-pandemic-in lgbt-peoples-mental-health/ (accessed May 16, 2022).
7. Panchal, Nirmita, et al. (2021), *The implications of COVID-19 for mental health and substance use*, Kaiser Family Foundation, https://www.kff.org/coronavirus-covid-19/issue-brief/the-implications-of-covid-19-for-mental-health-and-substance-use/ (accessed November 30, 2021).
8. Kaiser Family Foundation (2022), *Adults reporting symptoms of anxiety or depressive disorder during COVID-19 pandemic*, https://www.kff.org/other/state-indicator/adults-reporting-symptoms-of-anxiety-or-depressive-disorder-during-covid-19-pandemic (accessed May 14, 2022).
9. Panchal, Nirmita, et al. (2021), *The implications of COVID-19 for mental health and substance use*, Kaiser Family Foundation, https://www.kff.org/coronavirus-covid-19/issue-brief/the-implications-of-covid-19-for-mental-health-and-substance-use/ (accessed November 30, 2021).
10. Curtis, Sally, et al. (2021), *Provisional numbers and rates of suicide by month and demographic characteristics United States 2020, vital statistics rapid release*, U.S. Department of Health and Human Services, Center for Disease Control and Prevention, National Center for Health Statistics, Report No. 16, https://dx.doi.org/10.15620/cdc:110369 (accessed May 14, 2022), pp.2.
11. Hedegaard, Holly, et al. (2018), *Suicide mortality in the United States, 1999–2017*, NCHS Data Brief, No. 330, National Center for Health Statistics, Center for Disease Control and Prevention, https://pubmed.ncbi.nlm.nih.gov/30500324/ (accessed May 16, 2022), pp. 1–8.
12. Stone, Deborah, et al. (2021), Changes in suicide rates–United States 2018–2019, *Morbidity and Mortality Weekly Report*, 70, https://dx.doi.org/10.15585/mmwr.mm7008a1 (accessed May 16, 2022), pp. 261–268.
13. Ehlman, DC, et al. (2022), Changes in suicide rates—United States 2019–2020. *Morbidity and Mortality Weekly Report*, 71(8), https://dx.doi.org/10.15585/mmwr.mm7108a5 (accessed May 16, 2022), pp. 306–212.
14. Mental Health America (2023), *Self-injury (cutting, self-harm, or self-mutilation)*, https://www.mhanational.org/conditions/self-injury-cutting-self-harm-or-self-mutilation (accessed August).
15. Panchal, Nirmita, et al. (2021), *The implications of COVID-19 for mental health and substance use*, Kaiser Family Foundation, https://www.kff.org/coronavirus-covid-19/issue-brief/the-implications-of-covid-19-for-mental-health-and-substance-use/ (accessed November 30, 2021).

16. National Center for Health Statistics (2022), *U.S. overdose deaths in 2021 increased half as much in 2020—but are still up 15%*, Center for Disease Control and Prevention, https://www.cdc.gov/nchs/pressroom/nchs_press_releases/2022/202205.htm (accessed May 15, 2022).
17. Center for Disease Control and Prevention (2019), *Drug overdose deaths remain high*, U.S. Department of Health and Human Services, https://www.cdc.gov/drugoverdose/deaths/index.html# (accessed May 15, 2022).
18. Hedegaard, Holly, MD, et al. (2017), *Drug overdose deaths in the United States, 1999–2016*, National Center for Health Statistics, NCHS Data Brief, No. 294, https://www.cdc.gov/nchs/data/databriefs/db294.pdf (accessed May 16, 2022).
19. Scholl, L., et al. (2019), Drug and opioid-involved overdose deaths United States, 2013–2017, *Morbidity and Mortality Weekly Report*, 67(5152), https://dx.doi.org/10.15585/mmwr.mm6751e1, pp. 1419–1427.
20. Abramson, Ashley (2022), Children's mental health is in crisis, *American Psychological Association*, 53(1), https://www.apa.org/monitor/2022/01/special-childrens-mental-health (accessed May 15, 2022).
21. Panchal, Nirmita, et al. (2021), *Mental health and substance use considerations among children during the COVID-19 pandemic*, Kaiser Family Foundation, https://www.kff.org/blog/mental-health-and-substance-use-among-children-during-the-covid-19-pandemic (accessed May 16, 2022).
22. Center for Disease Control and Prevention (2022), *New CDC data illuminate youth mental health threats during COVID-19 pandemic*, U.S. Department of Health and Human Services, https://www.cdc.gov/media/releae/2022/p0331-youth-mental-health-covid-19.html (accessed May 14, 2022),
23. American Academy of Pediatrics (2021), *AAP-AACAP-CHA; declaration of a national emergency in child and adolescent mental health*, https://www.aap.org/en/advocacy/child-and-adolescent-healthy-mental-development/aap-aacap-cha-declaration-of-a-national-emergency (accessed May 14, 2022).
24. Keveney, Bill (2021), More young children are killing themselves: The COVID-19 pandemic is making the problem worse, UC Irvine School of Medicine, *USA Today*, https://www.choc.org/news.more-young-children-are-killing-themselves-the-covid-19-pandemic-is-making-the-problem-worse (accessed May 15, 2022).
25. Everett Jones, Sherry, PhD, et al. (2022), *Mental health, suicidality, and connectedness among high school students during the COVID-19 pandemic—adolescent behaviors and experiences survey, United States, January–June 2021*, United States Department of Health and Human Services, Center for Disease Control and Prevention, 71(3), pp. 16–21, pp. 19.
26. Charpignon, Marie-Laure, MSc, et al. (2022), Evaluation of suicides among adolescents during the COVID-19 pandemic, *JAMA Pediatr*, https://www/jamanetwork.com/journals/jamapediatrics/fullarticle/2791544 (accessed May 16, 2022),
27. Franklin, Michelle and LaFee, Scott (2021), *How adolescents used drugs during the COVID-19 pandemic*, UC San Diego Health, https://health.uscd/edu/news/releases/pages/2021-08-24/how-adolescents-used-drugs-during-the-covid-19-pandemic (accessed May 15, 2022).
28. Layman, Hannah, et al. (2022), *Substance use among youth during the COVID-19 pandemic: A systematic review, Curr Psychiatry Rep*, https://doi.org/10.1007/s11920-022-01338-z (accessed May 15, 2022).
29. Worldometer (2024), *COVID-19 data*, https://www.worldometers.info/coronovirus (accessed January 21, 2024).

30. Elflein, John (2022), *Number of new cases of COVID-19 worldwide from January 23, 2020 to May 8, 2022 by day*, Statista, https://www/statista.com/statistics/1103046/new-coronavirus-covid19-cases-number-worldwide-by-day (accessed May 15, 2022).
31. Elflein, John (2022), *Number of new cases of COVID-19 worldwide from January 23, 2020 to May 8, 2022 by day*, Statista, https://www/statista.com/statistics/1103046/new-coronavirus-covid19-cases-number-worldwide-by-day (accessed May 15, 2022).
32. International Committee of the Red Cross (2020), *World mental health day: New Red Cross survey shows COVID-19 affecting mental health of one in two people*, https://www.icrc.org/en/document/world-mental-health-day-red-cross-covid-19-mental-health-survey (accessed May 14, 2022).
33. World Health Organization (2022), Mental health and COVID-19: Early evidence of the pandemic's impact, *Scientific Brief*, https://www.apps.who.int/publications/i/item/who-2019-ncov-sci_brief-mental_health-2022.1 (accessed May 17, 2022).
34. Nochaiwong, Surapon, et al. (2021), Global prevalence of mental health issues among the general population during the coronavirus disease-2019 pandemic: A systematic review and meta-analysis, *Sci Rep*, 11, 10173, https://doi.org/10.1038/s41598-021-89700-8 (accessed May 17, 2022).
35. Fenollar-Cortes, Javier, et al. (2021), Gender differences in psychological impact of confinement during COVID-19 outbreak in Spain: A longitudinal study, *Front Psychol*, https://www.doi.org/10.3389/fpsyg.2021.682860 (accessed May 17, 2022).
36. Batterham, Philip, et al. (2022), Effects of the COVID-19 pandemic on suicidal ideation in a representative Australian population sample-Longitudinal cohort study, *J Affect Disorder*, 300, https://www.sciencedirect.com/science/article/pii/S0165032722000234#:~:text=This%20study%20found%20that%20the%20prevalence%20of%20suicidal,COVID-19%20pandemic%20in%20a%20representative%20Australian%20population%20sample (accessed May 17, 2022), pp. 385–391.
37. Schluter, Philip, et al. (2022), Patterns of suicidal ideation across eight countries in four continents during the COVID-19 pandemic era: Repeated cross-sectional study, *JMIR Public Health Surveill*, 8(1), e32140, https://pubmed.ncbi.nlm.nih.gov/34727524/ (accessed May 17, 2022).
38. Schluter, Philip, et al. (2022), Patterns of suicidal ideation across eight countries in four continents during the COVID-19 pandemic era: Repeated cross-sectional study, *JMIR Public Health Surveill*, 8(1), e32140, https://pubmed.ncbi.nlm.nih.gov/34727524/ (accessed May 17, 2022).
39. World Population Review (2022), *Suicide rate by country 2022*, https://www.worldpopulationreview.com/country-rankings/suicide-rate-by-country (accessed May 17, 2022).
40. Hoogte, Hollandse and Rozing, David (2022), *1,859 suicide deaths in 2021: 36 more than in 2020*, Contact with Statistics Netherlands, https://www.cbs.nl/en-gb/news/2022/17/1859-suicide-deaths-in-2021-36-more-than-in-2020 (accessed May 14, 2022).
41. Black, Lesly-Ann, Dr. (2021), *Suicide: Northern Ireland, Northern Ireland Assembly*, No. 23/21, NJAR 379-20, https://www.niassembly.gov.uk/globalassets/documents/raise/publications/2017-2022/2021/health/2321.pdf (accessed May 21, 2022), pp. 3.
42. Paul, Elise, et al. (2022), Factors influencing self-harm thoughts and behaviors over the first year of the COVID-19 pandemic in the UK: longitudinal analysis of 49,324 adults, *Br J Psychiatry*, (1), https://doi.org.10.1192/bip.2021.130, pp. 31–37.
43. Shrestha, Roshana, et al. (2021), Impact of the COVID-19 pandemic on suicide and self-harm among patients presenting to the emergency department of a teaching hospital in Nepal, *PLoS*

ONE, 16(4), e0250706, https://doi.org/10.1371/journal.pone.0250706. https://pubmed.ncbi.nlm.nih.gov/33930044. (accessed May 17, 2022).

44. Liem, Andrian, et al. (2022), Predicting self-harm and suicidal ideation during the COVID-19 pandemic in Indonesia: A nationwide survey report, *BMC Psychiatry*, 22(304), https://doi.org/10.1186/s12888-022-93844-w (accessed May 19, 2022). United Nations Office on Drugs and Crime (2021), *COVID-19 and drugs: impact outlook, World Drug Report 2021*, No. E.21.XL.8. pp. 11, 12, 49, 50, 52.
45. United Nations Office on Drugs and Crime (2021), *COVID-19 and drugs: impact outlook, World Drug Report 2021*, No. E.21.XL.8. pp. 11, 12, 49, 50, 52.
46. Peprah, Prince, et al. (2022), The correlates of substance use among older adults in Ghana during the COVID-19 pandemic, *Journal of Global Health Reports*, 6, e2022001, https://doi.org/10.29392/001c/31592. pp. 1.
47. Sylvestre, Marie-Pierre, et al. (2022), A longitudinal study of change in substance use from before to during the COVID-19 pandemic in young adults, *The Lancet Regional Health*, 8, 100168, https://doi.org/10.1016/j.lana.2021.100168 (accessed May 19, 2022).
48. World Health Organization (2021), *Opioid overdose*, https://www.who.int/news-room/fact-sheets/detail/opiod-overdose (accessed May 19, 2022).
49. United Nations Office on Drugs and Crime (2021), *COVID-19 and drugs: Impact outlook, World Drug Report 2021*, No. E.21.XL.8. pp. 63.
50. Imtiaz, Sameer, et al. (2021), The impact of the novel coronavirus disease (COVID-19) on drug overdose-related deaths in the United States and Canada: A systematic review of observational studies and analysis of public health surveillance data, *Substance Abuse Treatment, Prevention, and Policy*, 16(87), https://doi.org/10.1186/s13011-021-00423-5 (accessed May 19, 2022).
51. National Records of Scotland (2021), Drug-related deaths in Scotland in 2020, Crown, https://www.nrscotland.gov.uk/statistics-and-death/statistics/statistics-by-theme/vital-events/drugs/drug-related-deaths-in-scotland (accessed May 19, 2022).
52. Commonwealth Fund (2021), *Appendix exhibit 1 source notes death, European Drug Report 2021: Trends and developments*, https://www.commonwealthfund.org/sites/default/files/2022-05/baumgartner_intl_overdose_may-2022_appendix.pdf (accessed May 22, 2022).
53. UNICEF (2021), On my mind: Promoting, protecting, and caring for children's mental health, *The State of the World's Children*, https://www.unicef.org/yemen/media/5806/file/the-state-of-the-worlds-children-report.pdf (accessed May 21, 2022), pp. 100.
54. UNICEF (2020), *The impact of COVID-19 on the mental health of adolescents and youth*, https://www.unicef.org/lac/en/impact-covid-19-mental-health-adolescents-and-youth (accessed May 14, 2022).
55. Racine, Nicole, et al. (2021), *Global Prevalence of Depressive and Anxiety Symptoms in Children and Adolescents During COVID-19, JAMA Pediatric*, 175(11), 2482, https://pubmed.ncbi.nlm.nih.gov/34369987/ (accessed May 14, 2022), pp. 1142–1150.
56. United Nations (2020), *Policy brief: Impact of COVID-19 on children*, https://www.unsdg.un.org/resources/policy-brief-impact-covid-19-children (accessed May 22, 2022), pp. 1–3.
57. Xiao, Jiayi, et al. (2022), Impacts of psychological stress response on non-suicidal self-injury during the COVID-19 epidemic in China: the medication role of sleep disorders, *BMC Psychology*, 10(87), https://doi.org/10.1186/s40359-022-00789-6 (accessed May 19, 2022).

58. Corrigan, Claire, et al. (2022), Admission of children and adolescents with deliberate self-harm to intensive care during the SARS-CoV-2 out-break in Australia, *JAMA Netw*, 5(5) e2211692, https://pubmed.ncbi.nlm.nih.gov/35544133/ (accessed May 19, 2022).

59. Tang, Wen-Ching, et al. (2021), Prevalence and psychological risk factors of non-suicidal self-injury among adolescents during the COVID-19 outbreak, *Curr Psychol*, https://doi.org/10.1007/s12144-021-01931-0 (accessed May 19, 2022).

60. Zetterqvist, Maria, et al. (2021), A potential increase in adolescent non-suicidal self-injury during the COVID-19: A comparison of data from three different time points during 2011–2021, *Journal of Psychiatric Research*, 305, 114208, https://doi.org/10.1016/j.psychres.2021.114208 (accessed May 19, 2022).

61. UNICEF (2021), On my mind: Promoting, protecting, and caring for children's mental health, *The State of the World's Children*, https://www.unicef.org/yemen/media/5806/file/the-state-of-the-worlds-children-report.pdf (accessed May 21, 2022), pp. 38.

62. Odd, Todd, et al. (2021), Child suicide rates during COVID-19 pandemic in England, *Journal of Affective Disorders Reports*, 6, 100273, https://doi.org/10.1016/j.jadr.2021.100273 (accessed May 21, 2022).

63. Brown, Desmond (2021), *Number of youth in hospital after suicide attempt triple over 4-month period under COVID-19*, CBC News, https://www.cbc.ca/news/canada/hamilton/pandemic-safety-measures-childen-teen-health-impact-1.5953326 (accessed May 21, 2022).

64. Kim, Min-Jung, et al. (2022), *Changes in suicide rate and characteristics according to age of suicide attempters before and after COVID-19*, CHA Medical Center, 9(2), 151, https://doi.org/10.3390/children9020151 (accessed May 21, 2022).

65. Taylor, Alice (2022), *Suicide increasing amongst Europe's youth, governments underprepared*, EURACTIV, https://www.euractiv.com/section/coronavirus/news/suicide-increasing-amongst-europes-youth-governments-unprepaired (accessed May 21, 2022).

66. Taylor, Alice (2022), *Suicide increasing amongst Europe's youth, governments underprepared*, EURACTIV, https://www.euractiv.com/section/coronavirus/news/suicide-increasing-amongst-europes-youth-governments-unprepaired (accessed May 21, 2022).

67. Canadian Centre on Substance Use and Addiction (2021), *Mental health and substance use during COVID-19: Spotlight on youth, older adults & stigma*, https://www.ccsa.ca/mental-health-and-substance-use-during-covid-19 (accessed May 22, 2022).

68. Thung Sen, Lee, et al. (2021), Insights into adolescents' substance use in a low-middle-income country during the COVID-19 pandemic, *Front Psychiatry*, 14, https://doi.org/10.3389/fpsyt.2021.739698 (accessed May 22, 2022).

69. Mikwenha, Solomon, et al. (2021), *Increased illicit substance use among Zimbabwean adolescents and youths during the COVID-19 era: an impending public health disaster*, Society for the Study of Addiction, https://pubmed.ncbi.nlm.nih.gov/34729833/ (accessed May 22, 2022), pp. 1177–1178.

70. Grigoletto, Veronica, MD, et al. (2020), Rebound of severe alcoholic intoxications in adolescents and young adults After COVID-19 lockdown, *J Adolesc Health*, 67(5), https://www.ncbi.nlm.nih.gov/pmc/articles/PMC7490634/ (accessed May 22, 2022), pp. 727–729.

71. Columbia University Irving Medical Center (2021), *How does COVID affect mental health*, https://www/cuimc. columbia.edu/news/how-does-covid-affect-mental-health (accessed May 14, 2022).

72. Resnick, Brian (2021), *Psychiatrists are uncovering connections between viruses and mental health*, Voxmedia. https://www.vox.com/science-and-health/227883685/covid-19-depression-mental-health-risks-immunology (accessed May 23, 2022).

73. World Health Organization. (2020). *COVID-19 disrupting mental health services in most countries, WHO survey,* https://www.who.int/news/item/5-10-2020/covid-19-disrupting-mental-health-services-in-most-countries-who-survey (accessed November 30, 2021).
74. World Health Organization. (2020). *COVID-19 disrupting mental health services in most countries, WHO survey,* https://www.who.int/news/item/5-10-2020/covid-19-disrupting-mental-health-services-in-most-countries-who-survey (accessed November 30, 2021).
75. Centers for Medicare and Medicaid Services. (2021). *CMS data shows vulnerable Americans forgoing mental health care during COVID-19 pandemic,* https://www.cms.gov/newsroom/press-releases/cms-data-shows-vulnerable-americans-forgoing-mental-health-care-during-covid-19-pandemic (accessed November 30, 2021).
76. American Hospital Association (2022), *AHA house statement: America's mental health crisis,* February 2, 2022, https://www.aha.org/system/files/media/file/2022/02/aha-house-statement-ways-and-means-committee-americas-mental-health-crisis (accessed May 23, 2022).
77. J.L., Ayusi-Mateos *(*2021), Informing the response to COVID-19 in Spain: priorities for mental health research, *Rev Psiquiatr Salud Ment,* 14(2), https://doi.org/10.1016/j.rpsmen.2021.04.001, pp. 79–82.
78. D'Agostino, Armando, et al. (2020), Mental health services in Italy during the COVID-19 outbreak, *The Lancet Psychiatry,* 7(5), https://doi.org/10.101016/S2215-0366(20)30133-4 (accessed May 23, 2022).
79. Wiegand, Hauke, et al. (2022), Changes and challenges in inpatient mental health care during the first two high incidence phases of the COVID-19 pandemic in Germany—results from COVID psychiatry survey, *Front Psychiatry,* https://doi.org/10.3389/fpsyt.2022.855040 (accessed May 23, 2022).
80. Liu, Shuai, et al. (2020), Online mental health services in China during the COVID 19 outbreak, *The Lancet,* 7, https://doi.org/10.1016/S2215-0366(20)30077-8 (accessed May 23, 2022).
81. Zhong, Bao-Liang, et al. (2020), *Mental health problems, needs, and service use among people living within and outside* ncbi.nlm.nih.gov/33313137/ (accessed May 25, 2022).
82. National Center for Health Statistics (2022), *Household pulse survey,* Centers for Disease Control and Prevention, https://www.cdc.gov/nchs/covid19/health-care-access-and-mental-health-htm (accessed May 25, 2022).
83. Mental Health America (2021), *Mental health and COVID-19,* https://mhanational.org/mental-health-and-covid-19 (accessed May 26, 2022).
84. Mental Health America (2021), *Mental health and COVID-19,* https://mhanational.org/mental-health-and-covid-19 (accessed May 26, 2022).
85. American Hospital Association (2022), *AHA house statement: America's mental health crisis,* February 2, 2022, https://www.aha.org/system/files/media/file/2022/02/aha-house-statement-ways-and-means-committee-americas-mental-health- crisis,(accessed May 23, 2022).
86. Bandyopadhyay, Sohan, et al. (2020), Infection and mortality of healthcare workers worldwide from COVID-19: A systematic review, *BMJ Global Health,* 5(12), https://dx.doi.org/10.1136/bmjgh-2020-003-97 (accessed May 29, 2022).
87. Mehta, Sangeeta, et al. (2021), COVID-19: A heavy toll on healthcare workers, *The Lancet,* 9(3), https://doi.org/10.1016/S2213-2600(21)00068-0 (accessed May 26, 2022), pp. 226–228.
88. Mehta, Sangeeta, et al. (2021), COVID-19: A heavy toll on healthcare workers, *The Lancet,* 9(3), https://doi.org/10.1016/S2213-2600(21)00068-0 (accessed May 26, 2022), pp. 226–228.

89. Ghaleb, Yasser, et al. (2021), Mental health impacts of COVID-19 on healthcare workers in the Eastern Mediterranean Region: A multi-country study, *Journal of Public Health*, 43(3), https://doi.org/10.1093/pubmed/fdab321. pp. iii34–iii42.

90. Giannis, Dimitrios, et al. (2020), Impact of coronavirus disease 2019 on healthcare workers: Beyond the risk of exposure, *Postgraduate Medical Journal*, https://dx.doi,org/10.1136/postgradmedj-2020-137988 (accessed May 26, 2022).

91. Bandyopadhyay, Sohan, et al. (2020), Infection and mortality of healthcare workers worldwide from COVID-19: A systematic review, *BMJ Global Health*, 5(12), https://dx.doi.org/10.1136/bmjgh-2020-003-97 (accessed May 29, 2022).

92. Savage, Maddy (2020), *Coronavirus: The possible long-term mental health impacts*, https://www.bbc.com/worklife/article/20201021/coronavirus-the-possible-long-term-mental-health-impacts (accessed May 23, 2022).

Credits

Fig. 5.1a: Data Source: https://www.kff.org/coronavirus-covid-19/issue-brief/the-implications-of-covid-19-for-mental-health-and-substance-use/.

Fig. 5.1b: Data Source: https://www.kff.org/coronavirus-covid-19/poll-finding/the-impact-of-the-covid-19-pandemic-on-lgbt-people/#:~:text=Key%20Findings&text=Mental%20health%3A%20Three%2Dfourths%20of,(49%25%20v%2023%25).

Fig. 5.1c: Copyright © by Microsoft.

Fig. 5.2a: Source: https://www.cdc.gov/nchs/data/databriefs/db330-h.pdf.

Fig. 5.2b: Source: https://www.cdc.gov/mmwr/volumes/70/wr/mm7008a1.htm?s_cid=mm7008a1_w#suggestedcitation

Fig. 5.2c: Source: https://www.cdc.gov/mmwr/volumes/71/wr/mm7108a5.htm?s_cid=mm7108a5_w

Fig. 5.3a: Source: https://www.cdc.gov/nchs/data/databriefs/db330-h.pdf.

Fig. 5.3b: Data Source: Scholl L., et al, "Drug and Opioid-Involved Overdose Deaths — United States, 2013–2017," Morbidity and Mortality Weekly Report (MMWR), vol. 67, no. 5152. 2019.

Fig. 5.4: Data Source: https://www.worldpopulationreview.com/country-rankings/suicide-rate-by-country.

Fig. 5.5: Source: https://www.commonwealthfund.org/sites/default/files/2022-05/Baumgartner_intl_overdose_May_2022_Appendix.pdf.

Fig. 5.6: Source: https://unsdg.un.org/sites/default/files/2020-04/160420_Covid_Children_Policy_Brief.pdf.

Fig. 5.7: Data Source: Sohan Bandyopadhyay, et al., "Infection and Mortality of Healthcare Workers Worldwide from Covid-19: A Systematic Review," BMJ Global Health, vol. 5, no. 12, 2020.

Fig. 5.8: Data Source: Sohan Bandyopadhyay, et al., "Infection and Mortality of Healthcare Workers Worldwide from Covid-19: A Systematic Review," BMJ Global Health, vol. 5, no. 12, 2020.

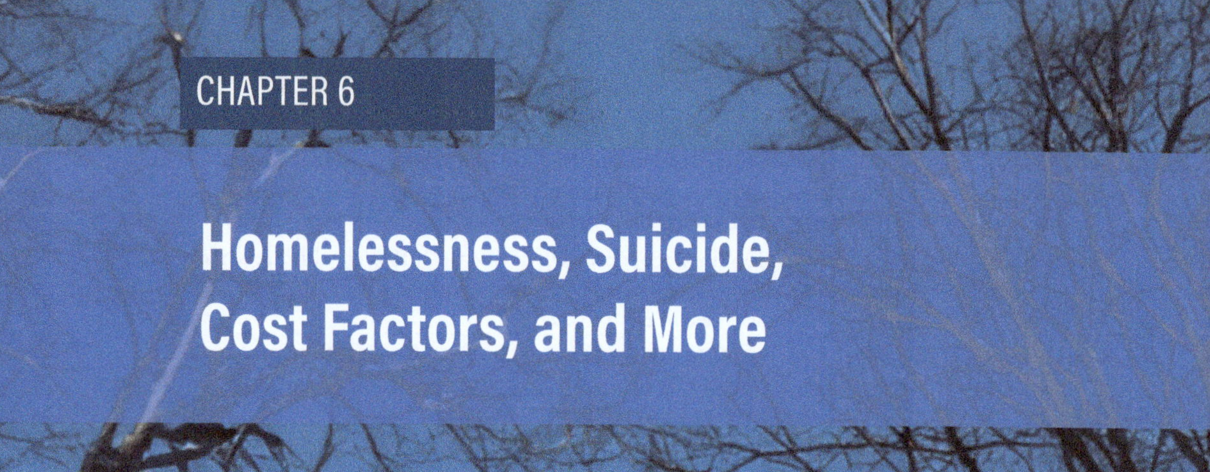

CHAPTER 6

Homelessness, Suicide, Cost Factors, and More

The main objective of this chapter is for the reader to realize there are some intrinsic and extrinsic adversities related to deinstitutionalization for mental health care recipients.

As previously discussed, the mental healthcare crisis has been identified as a global problem. There are several factors that have contributed to the lack of adequate behavioral and mental health services in many countries. These multifactorial dynamics have established ongoing research, data collection, interventions, and implementation of policies and procedures to attempt to decrease or eradicate these consequences for individuals needing mental health care.

Mental Health Care Adversities

In this chapter, we will explore several intrinsic and extrinsic components related to the crisis, including homelessness, cost factors, victimization, felony crime rates, community-based services, and noncompliance with treatment. Some of these viewpoints overlap with the perceptions of the positive reason basis for the deinstitutionalization process; thus, there are several different perspectives within society and the healthcare profession with regard to how to provide adequate mental health services worldwide.

Extrinsic Adversities

Extrinsic factors occur from social, governmental, and healthcare system processes. Recipients of mental health services generally have no control over these dynamics. As we continue to progress with deinstitutionalization globally, we must examine the issues of funding for community-based services and service fragmentation that is resulting in a significant number of individuals with serious mental illness ending up homeless.

Homelessness

Homelessness among individuals experiencing mental conditions has been increasing since the 1980s and is proving to be a significant consequence of the transition from institutional to community-based mental health care. A 2021 analysis of homelessness and mental illness concluded, "We found high prevalence of mental disorders among homeless people in high income countries, with around three-quarters having any mental disorder and a third having alcohol use disorders."[1] It is also becoming more and more recognized worldwide that homelessness can contribute to further mental health decline; it is not that deinstitutionalization generated homelessness, but more the way it has been implemented in many countries that sustains homelessness.

In 2022, it was estimated that there were approximately 72,888 individuals homeless (sheltered and unsheltered) with a serious mental illness in the United States.[2] When analyzing the ratio of homelessness to state population, California, Vermont, and Oregon had the highest rates in 2022. However, Washington, DC, had an estimated 65.8 homeless individuals per 10,000 people, which was significantly higher than any of the 50 states.[3]

As discussed previously, the shortage of psychiatric beds in the United States contributes to homelessness. An analysis in California revealed that the state had a shortfall of approximately 1,971 beds at the acute level (6.4 additional beds required per 100,000 adults) and a shortage of 2,796 beds at the subacute level (9.1 additional beds required per 100,000 adults)—or 4,767 subacute and acute beds combined.[4] Plus, the U.S. government spends approximately $35,578 per year for every person who endures chronic homelessness.[5]

Other Countries

It is estimated that between 30% to 35% of the homeless population in Canada have a mental illness, and 20% to 25% have a mental illness and misuse substances.[6] In 2020, the Organization for Economic Co-operation and Development estimated a total of approximately 900,000 people were experiencing homelessness in 21 European Union member states.[7] International studies conducted in the last 20 years have found lifetime prevalence rates for mental illness to be between 60% to 93% among the homeless.[8]

In Germany, data shows homeless people are affected by mental problems at a 3.8 times higher rate than the general population.[9] When individuals were interviewed by the organization FACIAM in Spain, it was reported that 70% of the homeless were at risk for having mental health decline, and 11.6% reported they had been diagnosed with a mental health problem.[10] A study cited by the Australian Institute of Health and Welfare found that 31% of homeless people experienced a mental health condition.[11] Figure 6.1 portrays homeless numbers per country in 2019.

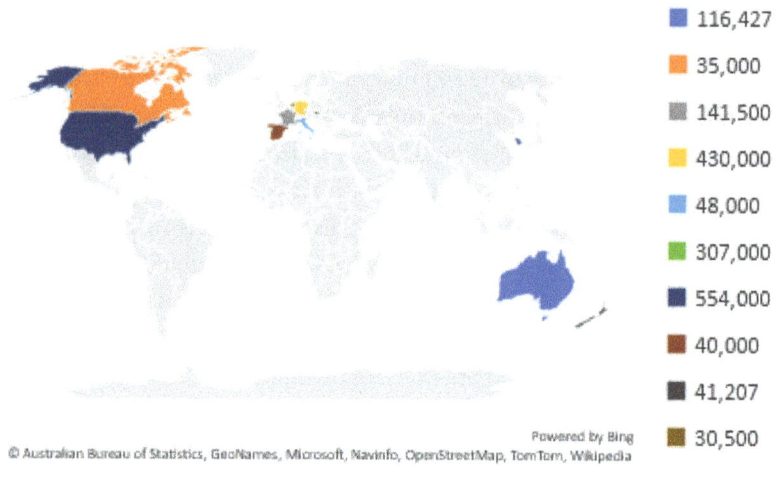

FIGURE 6.1 Homelessness Numbers by Country[15]

In 2021, the Institute of Global Homelessness estimated the homeless population in specific countries to be Germany 678,000; Iran 19,000,000; France 141,500; Spain 29,000; Italy 50,724; Greece 1,645; Iraq 3,300,000; Brazil 101,854; and Kenya 20,095.[12]

The Housing First Project, originally developed in New York, is a program that immediately provides homeless individuals with secure independent or communal housing. The program has been implemented in various forms in other countries, including Portugal, Denmark, the United Kingdom, Austria, Finland, France, Ireland, Hungary, Italy, Sweden, Belgium, Spain, and the Netherlands. A 2021 study found that the Housing First Programs decreased homelessness by 88% and improved housing stability by 41%.[13] An earlier study in Seattle, Washington, reported in 2018 that 90% of the individuals housed in their Housing First Project were still housed after one year versus 35% of the individuals who used the standard homeless interventions.[14]

There is an interplay between the lack of CMHCs, homelessness, and victimization; it is well-documented that lack of access to comprehensive, high-quality mental health care perpetuates and prolongs homelessness.[16]

Community-Based Services

Inadequate community mental health services contribute to a lack of treatment. SAMHSA reported in 2021, approximately 231 CMHCs existed in the United States.[17] In 2020, the total of other types of psychiatric care facilities available was psychiatric hospitals—668, outpatient mental health facilities—4,941, behavioral units in general hospitals—967, and day treatment facilities—429.[18] In 2022, the United States alone had 50 million adults who experienced a mental illness.[19]

It is reported that only about half of the CMHCs that were originally established for construction were actually built. Also, the funding to maintain these centers was not provided as originally planned. Thus, the Community Mental Health Act that was signed into law in 1963 was only partially successful because of the lack of construction of community-based mental health centers and the funding for community programs not being initiated or not existing for the long term. When evaluating the provision of mental health services, there is noted disparity in treatment and funding in comparison to medical health care services and the percentage of individuals who experience mental illness every year.

In 2021, WHO released *Guidance on Community Mental Health Services*, which promotes person-centered and rights-based approaches. The educational materials contain guidelines and best-practice examples from all over the world that include CMHCs, support groups and hospital-based services. WHO estimated that governments spend less than 2% of their overall health budgets on mental health care. Mental health service reform efforts worldwide are supported by their guidance.

Victimization

A study published in 2020 that evaluated victimization both inside and outside of the mental healthcare system revealed people with severe mental illness are vulnerable to becoming victims of violent and nonviolent crimes, as portrayed in Figure 6.2. It has been argued by some individuals that deinstitutionalization has increased the risk for individuals who experience serious mental illness of experiencing criminal acts in society because of homelessness. Some people perceive that institutionalization provides a safer environment versus the potential of clients living on the streets, where victimization could be very prevalent.

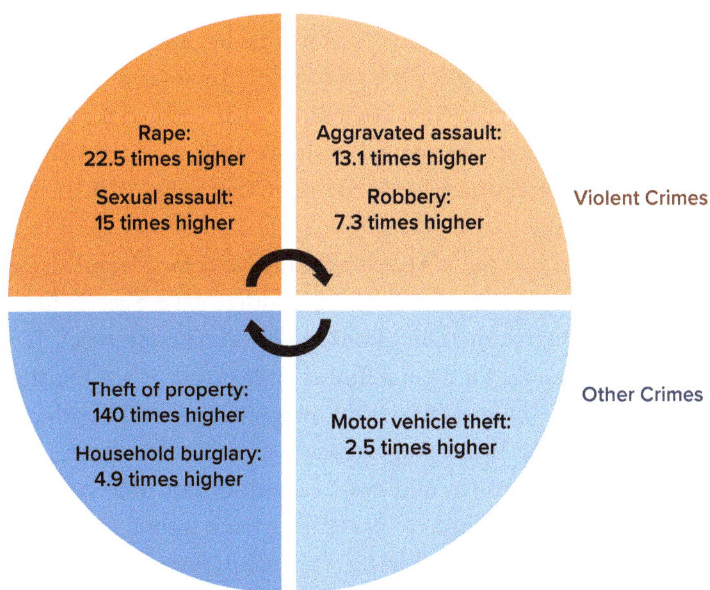

FIGURE 6.2 Mental Illness and the Likelihood of Victimization Outside the Hospital[22]

One study in 2020 revealed victimization outside of the mental healthcare system encompassed theft in 54.7% of the cases, 51.2% of the individuals reported physical violence without the utilization of a weapon, and sexual harassment occurred in 50.6% of the cases.[20] A 2006 study utilizing 16 randomly selected health agencies revealed that more than one quarter of the persons with serious mental illness had been victims of a violent crime in the past year, a rate more than 11 times higher than the general population rates.[21]

There are many different crimes that can be committed against individuals who experience serious mental illness, including theft, robberies, violent threats, physical abuse, aggravated assault, sexual violence, and coercive measures. With regard to the potential for homicide, a 2013 study revealed that individuals with a serious mental illness were at a fivefold increased risk of homicidal death.[23] Again, the majority of education on this subject matter reveals that individuals who experience mental illness are more likely to be victims of lethal violence than perpetrators and that interpersonal violence linked to mental illness has a very low probability rate.

The combination of mental illness, substance misuse, and potential poor physical health can make it difficult to maintain employment, residential stability, and deter the potential of being victims of violence. Improved community-based mental health services with implemented effective cost strategies could combat not only mental illness but homelessness as well.

Cost Factors

Studies reveal that approximately 72% of adults with a mental illness have at least one barrier to treatment, like cost or lack of needed insurance. There is variance in countries with regard to the affordability of mental health care for clients. In one survey, 15% of Americans revealed a lack of ability to obtain treatment; rates in France were at 21%, Norway at 16%, New Zealand at 7%, and the Dutch at 3%.[24] Spending in the United States on mental health treatment reached $225 billion in 2019.[25] It is estimated by the Lancet Commission that mental illness will cost the global economy $16 trillion by 2030.[26]

In 2019, WHO launched the WHO Special Initiative for Mental Health (2019–2023): Universal Health Coverage for Mental Health to ensure access to quality and affordable care for mental health conditions in 12 priority countries.[27] The aim is to increase treatment coverage for mental illness by ensuring access to mental health care over a 5-year plan. The reason base for integrating mental health care into all countries with universal health coverage is based on health and economic arguments. Figure 6.3 depicts populations (by millions) of countries with implemented universal health care. Again, the established connection between mental and physical health supports that with adequate mental health treatment, there could potentially be a reduction in physical health care costs. Plus, treating mental health decline early could reduce associated future mental health care costs.

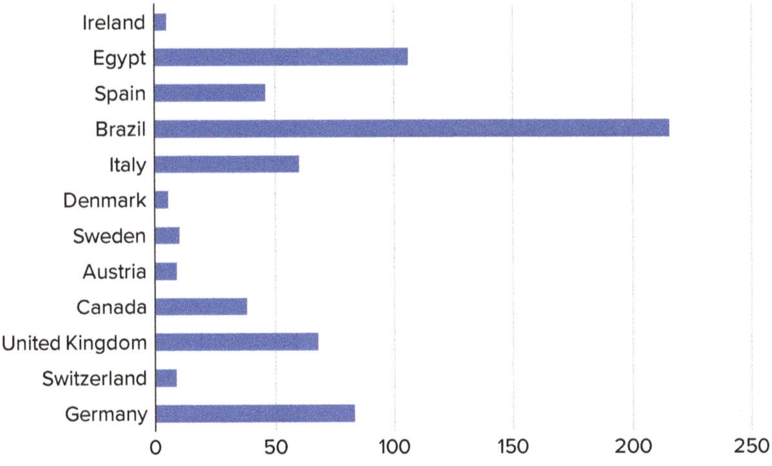

FIGURE 6.3 Population Countries With Universal Healthcare[28]

United States

The passage of the Affordable Care Act in the United States in 2008 legislated that insurance providers provide coverage for mental and behavioral health care, and the passage of the 2008 Mental Health Parity and Addiction Equity Act restricts insurance providers from behavioral and mental health coverage discrimination. Both processes have improved access to mental health services in America. Medicaid-managed care programs continue to be the largest payer for mental and behavioral health services in America.

Health care in the United States is currently a unique hybrid, multiple-payer system, but with elements of single-payer (i.e., Medicare, although beneficiaries also contribute through premiums), publicly subsidized private payers (e.g., employer-sponsored health insurance), socialized medicine (e.g., Department of Veterans Affairs, in which government is both the payer and the employer), and self-pay (i.e., out of pocket).[29]

Italy

Italy provides universal coverage through its National Health Service, which covers all citizens and legal foreign residents. It is funded by corporate and value-added tax revenues collected by the central government and distributed to the regional governments, which are responsible for delivering care. Residents receive mostly free primary care, inpatient care, and health screenings. Mental health services are provided, including CMHCs, community psychiatric diagnostic centers, general hospital inpatient wards, and residential/semi-residential facilities. Primary care is not involved in most Italian mental health treatment cases.[30]

Canada

Canadian Medicare is the universal health coverage in Canada. Health care is funded and administered primarily by the country's 13 provinces and territories. Each has its own insurance plan, and each receives cash assistance from the federal government on a per capita basis. Benefits and delivery approaches vary. All citizens and permanent residents, however, receive medically necessary hospital and physician services free at the point of use. Physician-provided mental health care is covered under universal insurance, and hospital-based mental health care is covered in general and psychiatric hospitals. Mental health has not been formally integrated into primary care.[31]

England

In England, all residents receive free public health care through the National Health Services (NHS), including mental health care; it is funded primarily through general taxation. As a governmental agency, NHS England, oversees and allocates funds to 191 Clinical Commissioning Groups, which govern and pay for care delivery at the local level.

Less serious illnesses—mild depression and anxiety disorders—are treated by general practitioners. The country has a program titled Increasing Access to Psychological Therapies, which integrates mental health into primary care. In 2017 and 2018, 550,479 people referred to the program completed an average of 6 weeks of therapy.[32]

France

Statutory health insurance (SHI) was extended over a 7-decade period to obtain universal health coverage in France. Coverage is compulsory and is provided to all residents by noncompetitive SHI funds. The insurance system is funded primarily by payroll taxes (paid by employers and employees), a national income tax, and tax levies on certain industries and products. SHI covers mental health care provided by general practitioners and psychiatrists in private practice, public mental health care clinics, and private psychiatric hospitals.[33]

Lack of adequate health insurance that covers mental health care and services can potentially lead to noncompliance with treatment and potential suicidal ideation.

Intrinsic Adversities

Intrinsic factors, generally, are related to some internal element that an individual might be able to improve or have some control over; they can include compliance with treatment and suicide.

Noncompliance with Treatment

Noncompliance with mental health treatments results in increased clinical, social, and economic costs. Without adequate supervision, many individuals who experience serious mental illness are noncompliant with medication management. It can evolve into a repeated cycle of the individual being stabilized on their medications, feeling that they are healed because of obtaining therapeutic dosage levels, and then thinking they no longer need their medications, so they stop taking them. Subsequently, they have to be rehospitalized and restabilized because of experiencing an acute relapse. Adequate community services that monitor medication compliance are a necessity in many psychiatric cases to maintain stabilization.

Adherence to psychiatric outpatient appointments in some studies has been shown to be associated with psychotherapy, regularly scheduling appointments, and lack of substance misuse, whereas noncompliance with appointments has been linked to poor insight, time, distance to travel, economics, and poor family support and/or therapeutic alliance. An individual's attitude toward their mental illness can also be a factor in compliance and noncompliance. Lack of education about specific psychiatric diagnoses, medication side effects and therapeutics, and benefits of adherence to scheduled appointments may contribute to perceived negative or poor attitudes about recovery.

Suicide Rates

Again, suicidal ideations are thoughts or ideas an individual experiences about terminating their life. There are both passive and active suicidal ideations. Passively thinking about suicide involves no longer wanting to live, and active suicidal ideation could involve forming a plan to die. Another estimate on suicide rates revealed every year, approximately 703,000 individuals commit suicide globally, and many more attempt suicide.[34] Figure 6.4 depicts suicide rates per region worldwide.

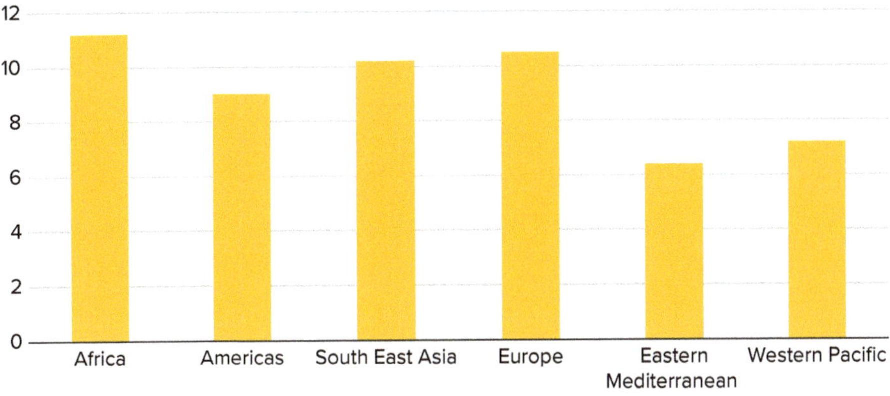

FIGURE 6.4 Suicide Rates by Region 2019 per 100,000 Population[37]

It is well established that there is a link between suicide and mental illness. From 2018 to 2019, there was a 2.3% decrease in suicides, and in 2020, the rate further declined by 3% in America.[35] In 2023, provisional estimates for suicide rates in the United States were released by the CDC, stating that rates increased by 5% in 2021, and in 2022, suicides increased from 48,183 deaths (2021) to 49,449 (2022) deaths.[36] Many more people attempt suicide; a suicide attempt is a clear indicator that something is extremely off balance in a person's life and serves as a risk factor for a successful suicide.

From 2014 to 2017, the number of CMHCs decreased by 14% nationally (from 3406 to 2920).[38] Suicide increased by 9.7% (from 15.4 to 16.9 per 100,000) in the same period.[39] A decline in CMHCs may be associated with 6% of the suicide increase, representing 263 additional suicide deaths.[40] It has also been established that the decline in hospital psychiatric beds could be partially attributed to increased suicide rates during this period. Since both psychiatric bed and CMHC numbers seem to keep decreasing in many countries, this could be attributed currently to adverse outcomes also.

Dr. Sharfstein (former American Psychological Association president) and colleagues argued in 2016 that the national U.S. suicide prevention strategy should include a necessary minimum number of psychiatric beds for patients at risk of suicide.[41] It has also been argued that there is conflicting evidence in relation to suicide rates and psychiatric bed availability. Italy has demonstrated a decline in suicides even with psychiatric bed reduction (1978, 7.1 suicides/100,000 population and 2006, 5.6 suicides/100,000 population).[42] Japan had the highest rate of suicides, with a 250 psychiatric beds/100,000 population ratio.[43] And the United Kingdom demonstrated results similar to Italy.[44] Christine Moutier, MD, states, "There is reason to believe that scaling up effective suicide prevention efforts in community and clinical settings can have a powerful preventative impact."[45] Stigma and discrimination of people facing mental health challenges can perpetuate further mental health decline, also potentially contributing to suicidal ideation and attempted suicides.

Stigma/Quality of Life

Stigma is defined as a negative and often unfair social attitude about a person, placing shame on them for a perceived deficiency or difference to their existence. Unfortunately, the stigma and discrimination associated with mental illness remain rampant worldwide. A lack of education and understanding of mental illness is one of the contributing factors to discrimination.

The adverse effects of stigma and discrimination, many times, subsequently lead to social isolation for individuals recovering from mental illness. This often, in turn, manifests increased symptomatology for people experiencing mental health conditions. The harmful effects of discrimination can include the following:

1. Shame, hopelessness, isolation
2. Bullying and harassment
3. Reluctance to seek assistance
4. Feelings of self-doubt

One study measuring attitudes toward mental illness found that only 25% of the people surveyed were sympathetic to mental health challenges.[46] These harmful effects of discrimination and stigma then decrease an individual's quality of life.

Several areas of a person's life that could be impacted by discrimination are employment, housing, long-term relationships, social life, economics, health care, and educational opportunities. Thus, an individual's overall quality of life is greatly diminished because of the exploitation, discrimination, and stigmatization associated with mental illness. The Center for Workplace Mental Health suggests organizations strive to "create a culture in which mention of depression, anxiety, post-trauma, and other common illnesses become as mentionable as diabetes, hypertension, and migraines."[47] A survey in 2018 found the first evidence of decreases in public stigma toward depression.[48]

Exploiting the mentally ill is not a new phenomenon; actually, it is highly prevalent in many countries. It is widely believed that exploitation is a form of abuse that involves a person being forced or coerced into situations that benefit others and entails sexual, financial, physical, and emotional forms. Some people believe that isolation and visibility of a person's mental condition lead to an increased probability of exploitation. The exploitation can be performed by family members, individuals in a community, medical service providers, employers, judicial personnel, and even those with religious affiliations. Erwin Goffman, author of *Stigma: Notes on the Management of Spoiled Identity*, stated, "There is no country, society, or culture where people with a mental illness have the same societal value as people without a mental illness."

BOX 6.1 A Critical Thinking Synopsis—Do You Agree?

The intrinsic and extrinsic adversities that have potentially been exacerbated with the deinstitutionalization process because of a lack of established community-based mental health services substantiates the need to improve mental health care systems globally, which will be elaborated on in the next two chapters.

Stigma, discrimination, and exploitation of people facing mental health challenges contribute to the deterrence of the recovery process; in the last chapter, it is pointed out by the U.S. government that the mental healthcare crisis is not a healthcare problem; it is a social problem.

Main Points

1. Homelessness among individuals experiencing mental conditions has been increasing since the 1980s and is proving to be a significant consequence of the transition from institutional to community-based mental health care.
2. It is reported that only about half of the CMHCs that were originally established for construction were actually built. Also, the funding to maintain these centers was not provided as originally planned.
3. WHO estimated that governments spend less than 2% of their overall health budgets on mental health care.
4. A study published in 2020 that evaluated victimization both inside and outside of the mental healthcare system revealed people with severe mental illness are vulnerable to becoming victims of violent and nonviolent crimes.
5. Studies reveal that approximately 72% of adults with a mental illness have at least one barrier to treatment, like cost or lack of needed insurance.
6. Noncompliance with mental health treatments results in increased clinical, social, and economic costs.
7. Unfortunately, the stigma and discrimination associated with mental illness remain rampant worldwide; a lack of education and understanding of mental illness are contributing factors.

Notes

1. Gutwinski, Stefan (2021), The prevalence of mental disorders among homeless people in high-income countries: An updated systematic review and meta-regression analysis, *PLoSMED*, 23, 18(8), e1003750, https://doi.org/10.1371/journal.pmed.1003750. https://www.ncbi.nlm.nih.gov/pmc/articles/PMC8423293/ (accessed September 20, 2022).
2. Statista Research Department (2023), *Mentally ill homeless people in the US by sheltered status 2022*, https://www.statista.com/statistics/962300/mentally-ill-homeless-people-in-the-us-by-sheltered-status (accessed August 22, 2023).
3. Statista Research Department (2023), *Mentally ill homeless people in the US by sheltered status 2022*, https://www.statista.com/statistics/962300/mentally-ill-homeless-people-in-the-us-by-sheltered-status (accessed August 22, 2023).
4. McBain Ryan, et al. (2022), *Adult psychiatric bed capacity, need, and shortage estimates in California—2021*, Rand Health Q, 9(4), https://www.ncbi.nlm.nih.gov/pmc/articles/PMC9519097/ (accessed August 22, 2023), pp. 16.
5. Roots Community Health Center (2021), *How much would it cost to end homelessness in America?*, https://rootsclinic.org/how-much-would-it-cost-to-end-homelessness-in-america (accessed October 30, 2021),
6. Blair, Nicole (2023), *Homelessness statistics in Canada*, https://madeinca.ca/homelessness-statistics-canada/ (accessed August 22, 2023).

7. Develtere, Patrick (2022), Data collection systems and homelessness in the EU—an overview, *European Journal of Homelessness*, 16(2), https://www.feantsaresearch.org/public/user/observatory/2022/EJH_16-2/EJH_16-2_RN2.pdf (accessed August 22, 2023), pp. 212.
8. FEANTSA (2023), *Homelessness is a health issue: A truly comprehensive European approach to mental health must consider the needs and access of people experiencing homelessness*, https://qqq.feantsa.org/public/user/PDFs FEANTSA_/Statement/FEA_statement_EC_communication_mental_ health_ comprehensive_approach_.pdf#:~:text=On%20the%207th%20of%20June%202023%2C%20the%20European,Regions%20on%20a%20comprehensive%20approach%20to%20mental%20health (accessed August 22, 2023).
9. FEANTSA (2023), *Homelessness is a health issue: A truly comprehensive European approach to mental health must consider the needs and access of people experiencing homelessness*, https://qqq.feantsa.org/public/user/PDFs FEANTSA_/Statement/FEA_statement_EC_communication_mental_ health_ comprehensive_approach_.pdf#:~:text=On%20the%207th%20of%20June%202023%2C%20the%20European,Regions%20on%20a%20comprehensive%20approach%20to%20mental%20health (accessed August 22, 2023).
10. FEANTSA (2023), *Homelessness is a health issue: A truly comprehensive European approach to mental health must consider the needs and access of people experiencing homelessness*, https://qqq.feantsa.org/public/user/PDFs FEANTSA_/Statement/FEA_statement_EC_communication_mental_ health_ comprehensive_approach_.pdf#:~:text=On%20the%207th%20of%20June%202023%2C%20the%20European,Regions%20on%20a%20comprehensive%20approach%20to%20mental%20health (accessed August 22, 2023).
11. Open Minds (2019), *The connection between homelessness and mental health*, https://www.openminds.org.au/news/the-connection-between-homelessness-and-mental-health (accessed November 20, 2021).
12. Institute of Global Homelessness (2022), *Better data project*, https://ighomelessness.org/global-homeless-data/ (accessed August 22, 2023).
13. National Alliance to End Homelessness (2023), *The case for housing first*, https://nlihc.org/sites/default/files/Housing-First-Research.pdf (accessed August 22, 2023).
14. Seattle School of Law (2018), *The effectiveness of housing first and permanent supportive housing*, https://www.law.seattle.edu/doc/5941324/the-effectiveness-of-housing-first-and-permanent-supportive-housing (accessed November 20, 2021).
15. Institute of Global Homelessness (2019), *State of homelessness in countries with developed economies*, https://docslib.org/doc/936328/state-of-homelessness-in-countries-with-developed-economies (accessed May 1, 2022), pp. 9, 10.
16. Bronxworks (2022), *Improving care coordination for homeless individuals with severe mental illness in NYC*, https://bronxworks.org/wp-content/uploads/2022/02/Improving-Care-Coordination-for-Homeless-Individuals-with-Severe-Mental-Illness-in-NYC-.8.2022.pdf#:~:text=The%20public's%20unease%20is%20driven%20primarily%20by%20encounters,high%20quality%20mental%20healthcare%20perpetuates%20and%20prolongs%20homelessness (accessed August 22, 2023). .
17. SAMHSA (2021), *SAMHSA awards record-setting $825 million in grants to strengthen community mental health centers, and support Americans living with serious emotional disturbances, mental illnesses*, https://www.samhsa.gov/newsroom/press-announcements/202109281153 (accessed October 30, 2021).

18. Michas, Frederic (2022), *Mental health facilities by type of facility in the U.S. 2020,* https://www.statista.com/statistics/712614/mental-health-facilities-by-type-of-facility (accessed May 1, 2022).

19. Mental Health America (2023), *Prevalence data 2022,* https://www.mhnational.org/issues/2022/mental-health-america-prevalence-data (accessed August 22, 2023).

20. Rossa-Roccor, Verna, et al. (2020), Victimization of people with severe mental illness outside and within the mental health care system: Results on prevalence and risk factors from a multicenter study, *Front Psychiatry,* 11:563860, https://www.frontiersin.org/articles/10.3389/fpsyt.2020.563860/full (accessed November 7, 2021), pp. 1–9.

21. Teplin, Linda, PhD, et al. (2006), Crime victimization in adults with severe mental illness, *Arch Gen Psychiatry,* 62(8), https://pubmed.ncbi.nlm.nih.gov/16061769/ (accessed November 7, 2021), pp. 911–921.

22. McBratney, Liz (2022), Victimization of people with mental illness, trauma and victimization, *Visions Journal,* 2007 3(3), https://www.heretohelp.bc.ca/victimization-people-mental-illness-vol3 (accessed May 2, 2022), pp. 8–9.

23. British Medical Journal (2013), *People with mental illness at highly increased risk of being murder victims, study suggests,* https://www.sciencedaily.com/releases/2013/130305200455.htm (accessed November 7, 2021).

24. Tikkanen, Roosa, et al. (2020), *Mental health conditions and substance use: Comparing U.S. needs and treatment capacity with those in other high-income countries, commonwealth fund,* https://doi.org/10.26099/09ht-rj07 (accessed November 7, 2021).

25. National Alliance on Mental Illness (2021), *What you need to know about the cost and accessibility of mental health care in America,* https://www.nami.org/press-media/in-the-news/2021/what-you-need-to-know-about-the-cost-and-accessibility-of-mental-health-care-in-america (accessed November 27, 2021).

26. The Carter Center (2018), Mental illness will cost the world $16 trillion USD by 2030, *Psychiatric Times,* 35(11), https://www.psychiatrictimes.com/view/mental-illness-will-cost-the-world-16-trillion-2030 (accessed November 27, 2021).

27. World Health Organization (2021), *Mental health: WHO special initiative for mental health,* https://www.who.int/initiatives/who-special-initiative-for-mental-health (accessed November 20, 2021).

28. World Population Review (2022), *Countries with universal health care 2022,* https://www.worldpopulationreview.com/country-ranking/countries-with-universal-health-care (accessed May 2, 2022).

29. Donnely, Peter, et al. (2019), Single-payer, multiple-payer, and state-based financing of health care: Introduction to the special section, *Am J Public Health,* 109(11), https://www.ncbi.nlm.nih.gov/pmc/articles/PMC6775924/ (accessed August 22, 2023), pp. 1482–1483.

30. Tikkanen, Roosa, et al. (2020), *International health care system profiles, Italy,* https://www.commonwealthfund.org/international-health-policy-center/countries/Italy (accessed May 2, 2022).

31. Tikkanen, Roosa, et al. (2020), *International health care system profiles, Canada,* https://www.commonwealthfund.org/international-health-policy-center/countries/Italy (accessed May 2, 2022).

32. Tikkanen, Roosa, et al. (2020), *International health care system profiles, England,* https://www.commonwealthfund.org/international-health-policy-center/countries/Italy (accessed May 2, 2022).

33. Tikkanen, Roosa, et al. (2020), *International health care system profiles, France,* https://www.commonwealthfund.org/international-health-policy-center/countries/Italy (accessed May 2, 2022).

34. Center for Disease Control and Prevention (2021), *Suicide prevention,* https://www.cdc.gov/suicide/index.html (accessed November 20, 2021).

35. Center for Disease Control and Prevention (2023), *Provisional suicide deaths in the United States, 2022,* https://www.cdc.gov/media/releases/2023/s0810-US-Suicide-Deaths-2022.html (accessed August 22, 2023).

36. Wikipedia (2019), *List of countries by suicide rate,* https://www.en.wikipedia.org/wiki/list-of-countries-by-suicide-rate (accessed May 3, 2022).

37. Kuntz, Leah, MD and Moutier, Christine, MD (2021), Breaking the trend: New CDC data on suicide, *Psychiatric Times,* https://www.psychiatrictimes.com/view/breaking-the-trend-new-cdc-data-on-suicide (accessed May 3, 2022).

38. Hung, Peiyin, et al. (2020), Changes in community mental health services availability and suicide mortality in the U.S.: A retrospective study, *BMC Psychiatry* 20, 188, https://doi.org/10.1186/s12888-020-02607-y (accessed November 28, 2021).

39. Hung, Peiyin, et al. (2020), Changes in community mental health services availability and suicide mortality in the U.S.: A retrospective study, *BMC Psychiatry* 20, 188, https://doi.org/10.1186/s12888-020-02607-y (accessed November 28, 2021).

40. Hung, Peiyin, et al. (2020), Changes in community mental health services availability and suicide mortality in the U.S.: A retrospective study, *BMC Psychiatry* 20, 188, https://doi.org/10.1186/s12888-020-02607-y (accessed November 28, 2021).

41. Williams, Benjamin (2020), *Q & A with former APA President Dr. Steven Sharfstein: Suicides and psychiatric beds,* https://psychiatryadvisor.com/home/topics/suicide-and-self-harm/qa-with-former-apa-president-dr-steven-sharfstein (accessed November 28, 2021).

42. Barbui, Corrado, et al. (2018), *Forty years without mental hospitals in Italy, International Journal of Mental Health Systems,* 12, Article number 43, https://doi.org/10.1186/s13033-018-0223-1 (accessed November 28, 2021).

43. Barbui, Corrado, et al. (2018), *Forty years without mental hospitals in Italy, International Journal of Mental Health Systems,* 12, Article number 43, https://doi.org/10.1186/s13033-018-0223-1 (accessed November 28, 2021).

44. Barbui, Corrado, et al. (2018), *Forty years without mental hospitals in Italy, International Journal of Mental Health Systems,* 12, Article number 43, https://doi.org/10.1186/s13033-018-0223-1 (accessed November 28, 2021).

45. Kuntz, Leah, MD and Moutier, Christine, MD (2021), Breaking the trend: New CDC data on suicide, *Psychiatric Times,* https://www.psychiatrictimes.com/view/breaking-the-trend-new-cdc-data-on-suicide (accessed May 3, 2022).

46. Newport Academy (2022), *Understanding mental health stigma and how we can create positive change,* https://www.newportacademy.com/ /resources/mental-health/teen-mental-health-stigma/ (accessed December 18, 2022).

47. American Psychiatric Association (2022), *Stigma, prejudice and discrimination against people with mental illness*, https://www.psychiatry.org/patients-families/stigma-and-discrimination (accessed December 18, 2022).

48. Pescosolido, Bernice, et al. (2021), Trends in public stigma of mental illness in the US, 1996–2018, *JAMA*, 4(12), e2140202, https://pubmed.ncbi.nlm.nih.gov/34932103/ (accessed December 18, 2022), pp. 1.

Credits

Fig. 6.1: Copyright © by Microsoft.

Fig. 6.1a: Data Source: https://www.un.org/development/desa/dspd/wp-content/uploads/sites/22/2019/05/CASEY_Louise_Paper.pdf.

Fig. 6.2: Adapted from Liz McBratney, "Victimization of People with Mental Illness: Barriers to Reporting Crime," Visions Journal, vol. 3, no. 3, p. 8. Copyright © 2007 by HeretoHelp.

Fig. 6.3: Data Source: https://worldpopulationreview.com/country-rankings/countries-with-universal-healthcare.

Fig. 6.4: Data Source: https://en.wikipedia.org/wiki/List_of_countries_by_suicide_rate.

PART III

AVENUES FOR IMPROVED MENTAL HEALTHCARE SERVICES

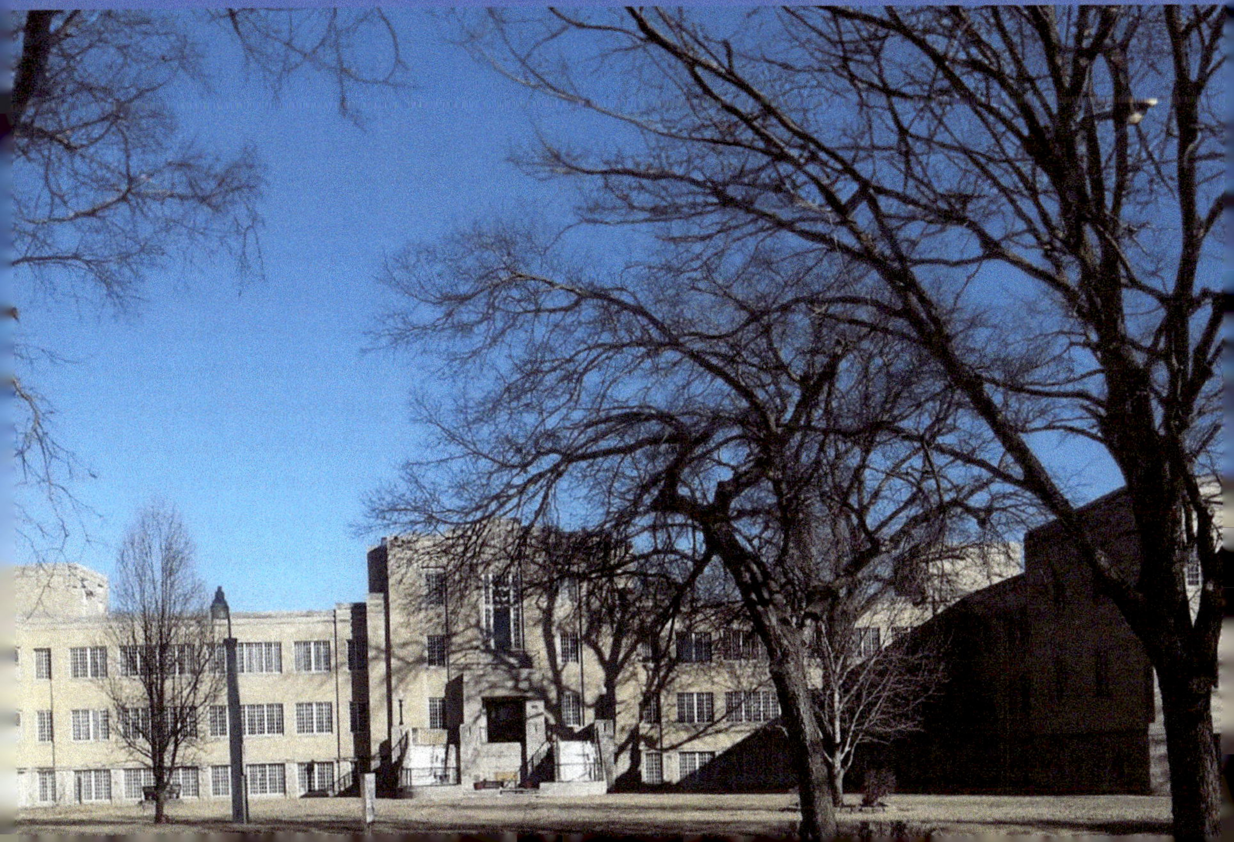

CHAPTER 7

Community Mental Healthcare Provisions

The main objective of this chapter is for the reader to be exposed to the balanced care and meta-community models related to mental healthcare delivery systems and protocols that establish efficient community-based mental health services.

The controversy about institutionalization versus community-based mental health services continues to elicit ongoing debate. As previously discussed, there are pros and cons presented on both sides of the dilemma. The interconnected dynamics discussed in previous chapters that have been potentially exacerbated by the deinstitutionalization process (homelessness, crime rates, cost factors, substance misuse, incarceration, and victimization) can be managed with effective community-based mental/behavioral health care services.

Globally, most countries are examining the mental healthcare crisis and attempting to implement interventions to resolve adversities and meet mental health care recipient's needs. The materials presented in this chapter cover community-based models and systems that could enhance mental well-being across the globe, including the meta-community and balanced care models that can assist in establishing recovery, stabilization, and crisis services worldwide. Implementation of the models and systems presented in this and the next chapter requires buy-in from communities, states, and governments to improve the mental well-being of each country's populace.

Many individuals perceive that we need both operational systems (community and hospital based) to adequately care for those experiencing mental illness to resolve the mental healthcare crisis. The balanced care model makes the case for both hospital and community-based mental health services to adequately meet the needs of those populations requiring psychiatric services.[1] The original model focuses on the integration of both general hospital and community-based services to ensure continuity of care. In most literature discussing this process, the mental health care provided is mainly community based, and general hospitals provide an important backup role. The model is based on a structured review of scientific evidence and is also informed by the experience of experts active in mental health system change in many countries worldwide.[2]

Yet, there are aspects to examine in this presented model, especially concerning lower income countries. It is suggested by some that if the model is to be globally used, adaptations should be instituted to facilitate the effectiveness of services delivered in lower and middle-income countries. Another model, the meta-community model, considers a broader range of services, such as social, housing, and homelessness services; justice; education; and employment. Following this holistic approach, the analysis of the mental health balance of care should not be restricted to just the hospital and community care.[3]

Mental Health Services

It is believed by many individuals that community-based mental health services are a more cost-effective approach to mental health treatment. Community mental health can be described as the principles and practices needed to promote mental health for a local population by (a) addressing population needs in ways that are accessible and acceptable; (b) building on the goals and strengths of people who experience mental illness; (c) promoting a wide network of supports, services, and resources of adequate capacity; and (d) emphasizing services that are both evidence-based and recovery oriented.[4]

The ability to live a fulfilling life is connected to an individual's mental health. Healthcare professionals need to be observant of the mental health crisis to assist in resolving adversities. Plus, advocates should work to change systems that perpetuate mental health problems and the improper treatment of individuals experiencing mental health challenges.

Community-based mental and behavioral health services are provided by governmental and county-operated organizations, as well as nonprofit and for-profit organizations. Stable housing is an ongoing problem for those individuals experiencing mental illness. For community-based mental health systems to function effectively, each community must include the provision of each client's housing needs, as housing is a basic need for recovery.

Housing

There are several options for community housing for those experiencing mental conditions. Each case should be assessed individually to meet each client's particular needs and abilities. Some individuals can function effectively with minimal to no supervision, while others require 24-hour assistance. There are several social services that can assist the mentally ill in finding appropriate housing, including RISE Services Inc., Catholic Community Services, and Mental Health America. Some of the options for housing are assisted living facilities, nursing homes, supervised group housing, partially supervised group housing, and supportive housing.

Assisted Living Facilities and Nursing Homes

These institutions provide a highly supervised and structured environment for individuals with severe mental illness. Staff is available 24 hours per day, 7 days per week, with licensed nurses available 24 hours per day in nursing homes. Assisted living facilities have nurses on call 24 hours per day and medication aides and/or certified nursing assistants on duty 24 hours per day. Independence and recovery are not the centered objectives of these facilities.

Supervised Group Housing

This type of housing facility provides the most support to individuals who experience mental illness, as it provides trained staff that are present in the home 7 days per week, 24 hours per day. Staff assist with activities of daily living such as medications, meals, paying bills, daily hygiene skills, transportation, and treatment programs. Supportive homes have measurable and impactful benefits (Harvard Health Publishing).[5] Statistics indicate that when living in supportive environments for the mentally ill, people

- spent 57% fewer days per year in a psychiatric hospital,
- made 58% fewer visits to emergency rooms, and
- had 50% lower rates for imprisonment.[6]

Partially Supervised Group Housing

Individuals residing in these types of settings do not require 24-hour-a-day assistance. Clients are able to perform their activities of daily living with minimal or no assistance. Some support is provided, but clients can be left unsupervised for several hours per day. Supervised and supportive housing integrate those with mental illness into the community, improving their quality of life.

Supportive Housing

Housing that is supportive in nature is one of the more independent living environments. Clients are able to complete all of their activities of daily living, but do have resources and people available if needed. Supportive environments usually encourage life skills and employment training for the client. Group therapy and counseling may also be a requirement to maintain a stable housing environment.

Homelessness Costs

A 2021 Annual Homeless Assessment Report in America found that more than 326,000 people experienced sheltered homelessness in the United States on a single night in 2021; the researchers conducting the study estimate that the cost of treating homeless individuals was $3.5 million or about $2,000 per person.[7]

According to the Canadian Alliance to End Homelessness, the cost of serving homeless people in Canada is high. In 2021, the cost for persons struggling with homelessness and mental illness was $53,144 per person.[8]

In the United Kingdom, evidence shows that people who experience homelessness for 3 months or longer cost an average of 4,298 euros per person for National Health Service services, 2,099 euros per person for mental health services, and 11,991 euros for a person in contact with the criminal justice system.[9]

A study in 2018 on supported housing consisted of 115 articles, evaluating mostly American populations, with smaller numbers considering Canadian, UK, Italian, Australian, and German contexts. This article revealed that the most robust evidence supports the effectiveness of the permanent supported accommodation model for homeless serious mental illness populations, specifically in generating improvements in housing retention and stability, in the appropriate use of clinical services over time, in reducing hospitalization rates, and in improving appropriate service use.[10]

Regardless of the client's housing needs and assistance levels, it is also imperative that communities provide the mental health care management needed for each individual, as it is also a necessity in stabilization, recovery, and maintenance.

American Community Mental Health Treatment

Once the housing dilemma is resolved for those experiencing mental illness, the provision of adequate treatment and recovery needs to be addressed. The current mental health systems implemented in most U.S. communities are not effective in serving the needs of many clients experiencing mental health challenges.

One analysis of meta-community mental health care (which encompasses housing and evidence-based practices) revealed that this model of care may be more reflective of the current state of mental health service provision and offer a better orientation in thinking about future service development.[11] Meta-community mental health care is consistent with the knowledge we already have of the principles of good mental health care, including the need for effective, accessible, efficient, and coordinated systems with meaningful service user participation and efforts to reduce the impact of stigma on access to care.[12] Many of the aspirations of community mental health care were founded on the recognition that mental illness can be caused, worsened, or maintained by damaging social processes in communities, neighborhoods, schools, and families. These social causes can be prevented, or their effects mitigated, by interventions that address the social toxins and by efforts to confront stigma and discrimination.[13]

In 1997, the Robert Wood Johnson Foundation, the Substance Abuse and Mental Services Administration, several state departments of mental health, and additional private foundations initiated a national demonstration to implement six specific evidence-based practices that were deemed essential community mental health services, including systematic medication management, assertive community treatment, supported employment, family psychoeducation, illness management and recovery, and integrated treatment for co-occurring disorders.[14]

Systematic Medication Management

Managing the medication regimen for those who experience mental conditions can seem like a daunting task. This process has been discussed briefly in a previous chapter, but we will elaborate in more detail at this time. The majority of adversity when dealing with this problem is the ever-evolving cycle of patients going off of their medications once they are stabilized. The author has personally seen this process unfold over and over again; the psychiatric hospital became a revolving door of patients being discharged and then readmitted after a period of time. This cycle emerges because clients feel better or have adverse effects from their psychotropic medications, thus perceiving they do not need or want their medications, and, subsequently, they quit taking the medications necessary to keep them stabilized.

In mental health cases, clients' not taking their medications as prescribed is widespread: between a third and a half of the people do not take their prescribed psychiatric medication at all, take less than the prescribed dose, or stop taking it abruptly.[15] An analysis of the reason base for clients' nonadherence to psychotropic medications revealed the following:

1. 55.6% was related to poor insight.
2. 36.1% was related to substance misuse.
3. 30.5% was related to negative attitudes toward medication.
4. 27.8% was related to medication side effects.
5. 13.4% was related to cognitive impairments.[16]

In China, a study on medication nonadherence revealed that among schizophrenia patients, bipolar disorder patients, and patients with major depressive disorder, nonadherence was approximately 56%, 48%, and 51% at the beginning of the 21st century.[17]

An intervention developed in the United States called "Common Ground" is a computerized recovery-oriented information and medication-related decision aid tool that has been associated with increases in self-reported overall health, perceived helpfulness concerning psychotropic medications, reductions in symptoms, and addressing concerns about negative medication side effects.[18] This system supports the process of shared decision-making with regard to mental health medication prescribing and utilization, which is being evaluated for potential enhancement of compliance.

Supported Employment

Stable employment is a contributing factor in recovery for those who experience mental conditions. Employment is key to social inclusion, and people with severe mental illness are still too often socially excluded and subject to stigma and negative attitudes regarding their contribution to society. It has been demonstrated that the majority of individuals who have a mental illness or a co-occurring disorder want to work, yet face many challenges attempting to obtain or sustain employment.

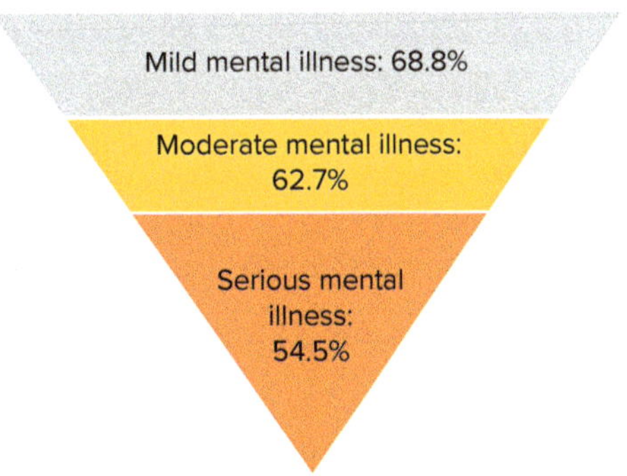

FIGURE 7.1 Mental Illness Percentage Rate Decreasing for Employment[22]

Research demonstrates that employment rates for individuals receiving mental health services range from 17.9% to 39%, and only 2% of adults with SMI have access to supported employment.[19] A 2021 analysis of patients with SMI aged 18–65 years who were interviewed by trained staff using standardized instruments, analyzing the relationship between potential predictors and a strong preference for employment using a hierarchic binary logistic regression model, revealed only about one quarter (27.9%) of SMI patients were in competitive employment, another quarter were unemployed (25.9%).[20] Figure 7.1 illustrates the decreasing percentage rate for employment encompassing mental illness.

Supported employment (SE) is defined as competitive work in integrated work settings or employment in integrated work settings in which individuals are working toward competitive work consistent with the strengths, resources, priorities, concerns, abilities, capabilities, interests, and informed choices of the individuals. Individuals with the most significant disabilities may qualify and benefit from SE, including individuals

1. for whom competitive employment has not traditionally occurred,
2. for whom competitive employment has been interrupted or intermittent as a result of a significant disability, and
3. for whom, because of the nature and severity of their disability, need intensive SE services for a period and any qualified extension.[21]

Sustained employment for those who experience mental illness assists in decreasing poverty, unemployment rates, homelessness, Medicaid utilization, and societal stigma. Plus, it helps those experiencing mental illness to maintain health insurance, increase their self-esteem, and establish social systems to eradicate isolation. SAMHSA developed the Individual Placement and Support (IPS) model, an evidence-based practice specifically for individuals with serious mental illness. The IPS model is based on core principles that include the following:

- Every consumer/client who wants to work is eligible.
- Competitive jobs are the primary goal of SE.
- SE services are integrated with comprehensive mental health treatment.

- Personalized benefits counseling is provided to every consumer/client.
- Job placement happens when the individual believes they are ready.
- Employment specialists (job coaches) receive extensive training in SE and developing relationships with businesses and other employment opportunities.
- Consumers/clients receive job support for as long as required.[23]

In Tennessee, IPS is an evidence-based model of SE that helps individuals living with mental health, substance use, and/or co-occurring disorders find and maintain competitive employment. IPS started in Tennessee in 2013 with four pilot sites and has expanded to 14 different providers with more than 30 different IPS teams supporting different populations. Nationally, across 28 randomized control trials, IPS showed a competitive employment rate of 55% compared to 25% with other SE models. Creating a jobs initiative through monetary assistance in 2023 allowed the state to expand the number of people served by about 740 individuals.[24]

An analysis in 2023 regarding SE and IPS examined 28 studies on IPS, four other IPS studies that were augmented by another intervention, and 24 other forms of supported employment. The studies ranged from under 10 to 173,000 participants, with time horizons from 6 weeks to 50 years. Other than one economic evaluation of a six-country trial in Europe, all were single-country studies. In total, 17 (31%) were set in the United Kingdom, 18 (33%) in the United States, and eight (15%) in the Nordic countries. The conclusion was there is a strong economic case for the implementation of SE and individual placement support programs.[25]

Family Psychoeducation

Described as a method-based practice established on clinical findings, family psychoeducation is used to train and educate families to work with mental health professionals as a part of clinical treatment for those who experience mental illness. The major goal in this process is to improve client outcomes (recovery), prevent relapses, and assist family members in developing positive coping skills. Psychoeducation can be incorporated for the individual, family members, and/or friends and can be structured individually or in groups. The major psychoeducational models can be categorized into four approaches:

1. Informational Model: The emphasis of this model is to provide families the knowledge about psychiatric illness and its management. The aim of this approach is to improve the families' awareness of the illness and contribution to the management of the client.
2. The Skill Training Model: This model is directed at systematically developing specific behaviors so that family members can enhance their capacity to assist ill relatives and manage the illness more effectively.
3. The Supportive Model: It is an approach that generally uses support groups designed to engage the families of patients in sharing their feelings and

experiences. Here, the main goal is to enhance and improve the emotional capacities of the families to cope with caring for their ill relatives.

4. Comprehensive Model: It is also called the combination approach because it consists of information, skill training, and the supportive model. In the initial phase of this approach, members are given lectures about the illness. They are also to take part in a multifamily support group. In the final phase, they have to participate particularly as a member in individual sessions with a mental health professional.[26]

The Cochrane Schizophrenia Group conducted a study on brief (10 sessions or less) psychoeducation benefits with the following data obtained:

- Participants receiving brief psychoeducation were less likely to be noncompliant with medication regimens.
- Relapse rates were significantly lower among participants receiving brief psychoeducation (decreased hospital readmission).
- Brief psychoeducation can improve the long-term global state, promote improved mental state in short-term and medium-term periods (increased satisfaction with mental health services), and lower the incidence and severity of anxiety and depression.
- Improved social function, such as rehabilitation status and social disability (improved quality of life).[27]

A recent analysis of 85 research studies revealed psychoeducation should be an early intervention in those newly diagnosed with schizophrenia because of its evidence-based benefits.[28] Another recent systematic review of 20 studies concluded that psychoeducation appeared to reduce relapse and promote adherence in severe mental illnesses such as schizophrenia.[29] Despite recommendations in clinical practice guidelines, family psychoeducation is not widely available throughout the world.[30]

Illness Management and Recovery

Instituting an Illness Management and Recovery (IMR) Program assists clients in learning about mental illness and treatment strategies, decreasing symptoms, reducing relapses and hospitalizations, and progressing toward recovery. The programs typically consist of 3 to 10 weeks of weekly or biweekly sessions, with the client working with a trained practitioner. The core components of the program are behavior tailoring, psychoeducation, relapse prevention, and coping skills training.[31]

Management of symptoms and recovery can have different meanings for individuals. What the author, as a nurse, perceives as being in recovery or recovering from a psychiatric condition could be totally incorrect for another person. It is crucial that each person is allowed to identify their own goals, steps, and strategies to obtain what they feel is recovery. There are different interventions to be used to assist in mental health recovery, including the following:

- Self-help programs
- Support systems
- Making time for leisure
- Spirituality
- Staying active
- Maintaining physical health
- Following treatment strategies
- Being cognitive of the environment
- Creativity[32]

Setting, pursuing, and achieving goals also assists in recovery from mental conditions. Each individual needs to identify their own goals and objectives to obtain those ambitions; it is rare that two individuals would identify with the same perceptions of what is important or has meaning for them in life.

Prevention of relapse is also an important aspect of healing; it acknowledges past triggers, early warning signs, support, and interventions for early warning signs.[33] Self-management is an important aspect of this process. Managing stress is a major part of wellness, each individual needs to be able to identify stressful situations and manage those situations to enhance quality of life.

Obtaining optimal well-being is possible after experiencing mental illness, as demonstrated in a recent Canadian study illustrated in Figure 7.2. Compared with 24.1% of participants without a history of psychopathology, 9.8% of participants with a lifetime history of psychopathology met optimal well-being.[34]

The IMR Program has been implemented in various other countries, including the Netherlands, Denmark, Norway, Sweden, Spain, Japan, and Singapore.[36] A study analyzing 187 outpatients over an 18-month period, comprising 12 months

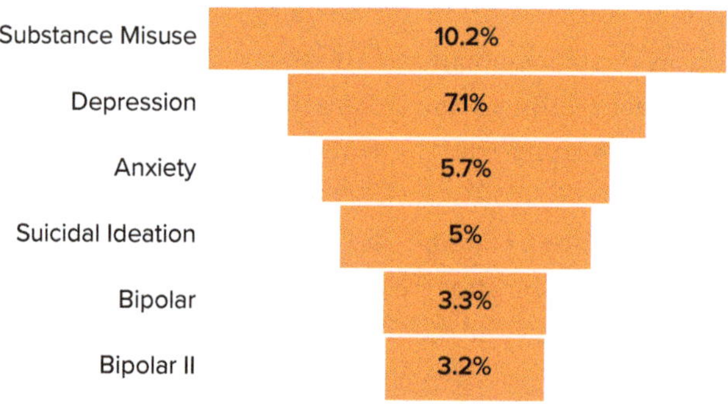

FIGURE 7.2 Mental Illness and Optimal Well-Being[35]

of treatment and 6 months of follow-up, demonstrated that patients who received IMR showed statistically significant improvement in self-reported overall illness management (the primary outcome). Moreover, they showed an improvement in self-esteem, which is a component of personal recovery. Patients showed statistically significant improvement in clinician-rated overall illness management, social support, clinical and functional recovery, and self-stigma over time. IMR completion was associated with stronger effects. High IMR fidelity was associated with self-esteem. This study confirms the efficacy of IMR in overall illness self-management.[37]

Integrated Treatment for Co-occurring Disorders

As briefly discussed earlier, this treatment model focuses on providing services that are tailored to address both mental illness and substance misuse concurrently for dual-diagnosed individuals. There are four stages of treatment encompassed in the process:

1. Engagement—assertive outreach to engage and retain
2. Persuasion—develop trust
3. Active treatment—motivational interventions: education, support, counseling, psychotherapy, psychopharmacology
4. Relapse prevention—stress management, social networks, medication management, coping skills[38]

It also involves the utilization of multiple treatments, such as the combination of psychotherapy and pharmacotherapy. Again, integrated treatment for comorbidity has been found to be consistently superior compared to treatment of individual conditions with separate treatment plans.[39] One such treatment model is integrated group therapy, developed by McLean's Roger D. Weiss, MD; several randomized clinical trials have shown this is a highly effective treatment.[40] Studies reveal that only 25% of behavioral health agencies offer integrated care, and below 7% of individuals who need integrated services receive it.[41]

Assertive Community Treatment

Assertive community treatment (ACT) is a multidisciplinary team approach with assistive outreach in the community for individuals with severe mental illness who are at risk for psychiatric crisis, hospitalization, and involvement with the criminal justice system. Team members are trained in the areas of psychiatry, social work, nursing, substance misuse, and vocational rehabilitation. The goal is to assist clients with living independently in the community (in their homes) and to assist families with their care. It is estimated that only six states have implemented the ACT program statewide. Effective July 1st, 2023, the South Carolina Department of Health and Human Services will cover ACT services through the Medicaid State Plan.[42] ACT has also been implemented in Canada, Australia, and the United Kingdom.

American Community Mental Health Centers/ Programs

Between the years of 1947 and 1951, there was initiation of the first community-based mental health services in the United States. The Health Amendments Act of 1956 authorized support of community services, initiating halfway houses, daycares, and aftercare programs for those experiencing mental illnesses in the nation. In this section, we will discuss CMHCs, Certified Community Behavioral Health Clinics (CCBHCs), day programs, Federally Qualified Health Centers (FQHCs), clinical residential treatment programs, and funding/cost-effectiveness related to mental health care provisions.

Again, the Community Mental Health Centers Act emphasized the development of community-based facilities to provide continuity of care, including prevention, treatment, and rehabilitation. Numbers were provided on the available CMHCs in previous chapters; additionally, CCBHCs were also established in 2014; these facilities offer mental health and substance use services to individuals. According to the SAMHSA, there are over 500 CCBHCs operating across the country as either CCBHC-E grantees, as clinics participating in their state's Medicaid demonstration, or as a part of independent state CCBHC programs.[43]

SAMHSA has a section 223 Demonstration Program for CCBHHCs; the program assists states in establishing CCBHCs, creating a 2-year demonstration program for states to certify community behavioral health clinics. In 2015, 24 states received planning grants to help them prepare for the demonstration program. In 2020, Congress expanded the program to Michigan and Kentucky.

There were ten states participating in the demonstration in 2022: Kentucky, Michigan, Minnesota, Missouri, New York, New Jersey, Nevada, Oklahoma, Oregon, and Pennsylvania. CCBHCs are required to offer a broad array of coordinated, evidence-based services. CCBHCs must provide 24/7 mobile crisis teams and crisis stabilization; screening, assessment, and diagnosis; patient-centered treatment planning; outpatient mental health and substance use services; primary care screening and monitoring of key health indicators; targeted case management; psychiatric rehabilitation services; peer and family supports; and tailored mental health care for members of the armed forces and veterans.[44] In March of 2023, 15 additional states received planning grants.

Federal Qualified Health Centers

FQHCs are important safety net providers in rural areas. FQHCs are outpatient clinics that qualify for specific reimbursement systems under Medicare and Medicaid. FQHCs serve an underserved area or population and offer a sliding fee scale, providing a variety of health services (these clinics are not specifically focused on mental health care) that include mental health and substance misuse services. There are 1,403 official FQHC locations in the United States.[45]

Funding and Cost-Effectiveness

The Community Mental Health Services Block Grant program makes funds available to all 50 states. The funds can be used for new programs or to supplement existing programs. In 2021, SAMSHA awarded $825 million in grants to 231 CMHCs to strengthen services provided. It is estimated that CMHCs have a significant impact on cost savings, with an estimated $10 per day expenditure for community-based mental health treatment. Whereas other mental illness treatment options, such as a state psychiatric hospital, average $428 per day.[46] Again, WHO implemented a new guidance on community mental health services promoting person-centered and rights-based approaches that further affirm that mental health care must be grounded in a human-rights-based perspective, and the guidance is recommended by the WHO Comprehensive Mental Health Action Plan of 2020–2030.[47]

Day Programs

Day programs assist in recovery from mental illness through education, developing strengths, and building skills. Services usually focus on socialization, self-advocacy, development of support, recovery, and community living skills. Psychosocial rehabilitation can include self-management of mental and physical health conditions, independent living skills, and psychiatric rehabilitation. Typically, the programs are 3 to 5 hours, 3 to 5 days a week, with a duration of 12 to 20 weeks.

Clinical Residential Treatment Programs

In clinical residential treatment programs, individuals with mental illness reside at the treatment center. It provides more of a home-like atmosphere versus a hospital. This process provides a more intense level of care, as staff are available 24 hours/day and 7 days/week. The programs provide a holistic approach to stabilization and recovery. Many times, an individual needs to leave the environment they currently are engaged with in order to progress effectively in recovery. Residential treatment programs offer individuals with difficult living environments an alternative to healing. Typically, these programs can last 30 days to 12 months. Figure 7.3 illustrates residential treatment facilities in the United States.

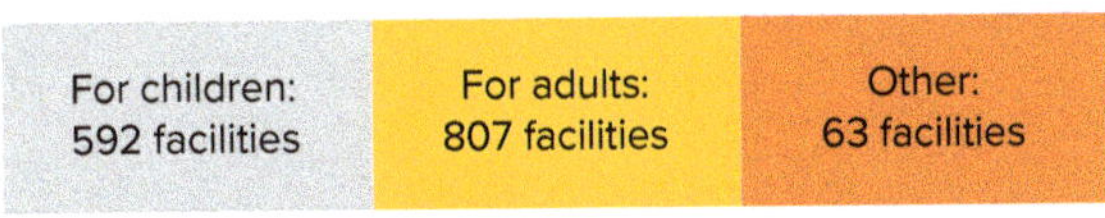

FIGURE 7.3 Residential Treatment Facilities in the United States[48]

Global Perspective: Community Mental Health Services

The community-based model in Peru was initiated with a series of reforms supported by advocacy from the Ombudsperson's Office that established mental health care coverage in the national health insurance, developed a budget program for mental health, and passed a new mental health law. These actions resulted in an increase in community-based mental health centers from 22 facilities in 2015 to 203 facilities in 2021. There are also 30 behavioral service units in general hospitals and 48 halfway houses in this country.[49]

Serbia

Mental health reform in Serbia began in 2007 with the National Strategy for Development of Mental Health Care. Five mental health centers (centri za mentalno zdravlje) were opened in 2019. The focus of the new strategy in Serbia is the reorganization of the network of psychiatric institutions, strengthening psychiatric services in general hospitals, and gradual reduction of the number of beds in large hospitals and the number of patients in institutions.[50]

Turkey

In 2006, a community mental health program was established in Turkey. The country currently has 177 community health centers affiliated with state hospitals, mostly focused on adult patients with schizophrenia and mood disorders. There has also been a reduction of in-patient mental health beds. Implementation of other services for specific populations, such as the National Action Plan for individuals with Autism Spectrum Disorder, has been developed in this country.[51]

Mexico

Community mental health services in Mexico are provided through the Comprehensive Mental Health Centers. There are 54 current centers in Mexico that provide short- and long-term stays. The circumstances in Mexico are that the distribution of human resources and mental health care are centralized in the main cities, and a large population is left at a disadvantage. The average access time to the nearest mental health center for some populations exceeds 30 minutes and reflects that access to mental health care is well beyond what is expected, generating an extra risk for psychiatric emergencies.[52]

Italy

It is believed by some individuals that Trieste, Italy, has been very successful in the implementation of community-based mental health care services, and the country of

Italy has outperformed other countries with the closing of state funded psychiatric institutions. The Mental Healthcare Centers in Italy provide overnight and daytime hospitality, outpatient services, home visits, personalized and family therapeutic work, group activities, rehabilitation and prevention interventions, support for rights, home support, and consultation services. The Department of Mental Health in Italy places a great emphasis on working with the wider community, encouraging a viewpoint that encompasses promoting mental health and taking care of the social fabric.[53] It has also been reported that the homelessness of those experiencing mental illness is not as extensive in Italy as in other countries. Community crisis intervention modalities are a necessity in all countries to establish effective mental health services.

Health Teams to Address Community Crisis Intervention

Mobile crisis health teams have been implemented in some areas in the United States. Mental health professionals respond to crisis or emergency situations, assisting to decrease psychiatric hospitalizations, stabilize the client, and decrease imprisonment. It has been identified that the benefits of crisis teams include stabilization of mental health, improved safety, suicide prevention, family support, increased navigation with services, and cost-effectiveness.

The NAMI recommends that every community implements a crisis team and has listed three core elements: regional or statewide 24/7 crisis call centers, mobile crisis teams, and crisis receiving and stabilization programs. Crisis receiving and stabilization services should provide recovery-focused, trauma-informed, and "living-room-like" crisis observation and stabilization.[54] NAMI reports that crisis intervention teams exist in 2,700 communities nationwide.[55]

SAMHSA has released a document called "National Guidelines for Behavioral Health Crisis Care Best Practice Toolkit," which provides guidance on how to improve crisis response. The toolkit includes distinct sections for defining national guidelines in crisis care, tips for implementing care that aligns with national guidelines, and tools to evaluate the alignment of systems to national guidelines.

SAMHSA recommends that states and territories use the Mental Health Block Grant supplemental funding from the Bipartisan Safer Communities Act to, among other things, develop statewide mental health emergency preparedness and response plans focused on collaboration with law enforcement and other local agencies, identify mobile crisis teams that can be deployed rapidly throughout the state to address mental health during an emergency, provide behavioral health crisis response trainings to agencies and providers, identify culturally and linguistically appropriate support for diverse populations, and build and leverage relationships with 988 Suicide and Crisis Lifeline call centers, child welfare organizations, schools, and others.[56]

The 988 number mental health crisis hotline implemented on July 16th, 2022, to provide 24/7 phone, chat, or text support to individuals experiencing a mental health crisis or in need of suicide prevention services will hopefully help to assist in decriminalizing mental health. The hotline can assist in mobilizing a crisis team if needed, thus decreasing law enforcement involvement in mental health emergencies. Figure 7.4 depicts the number of contacts to 988 since implementation.

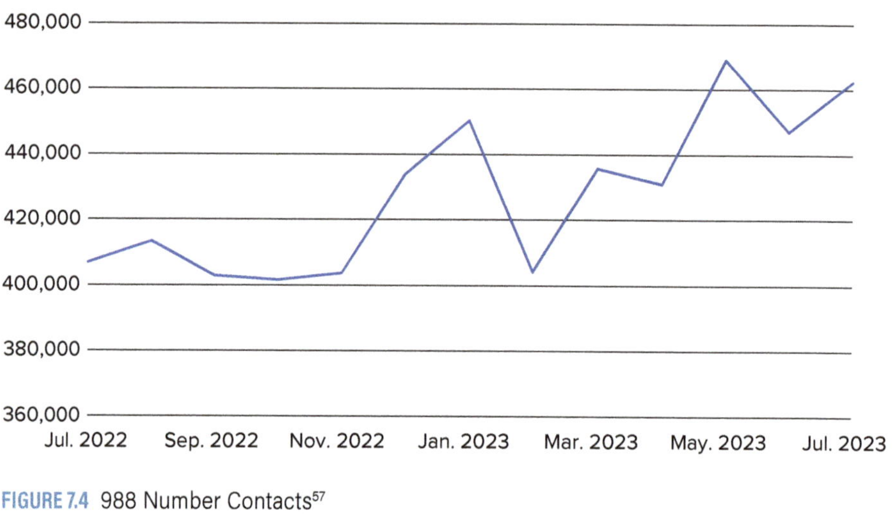

FIGURE 7.4 988 Number Contacts[57]

It is believed by some mental health professionals that the 988 number holds the promise of equitable health care response to a health care issue with better outcomes as individuals receive the services and support they need to remain in their communities and thrive.

Vancouver, Canada, developed Car 87, the country's oldest police mental health crisis response initiative. The Car 87 team consists of one Vancouver police constable and a psychiatric nurse to provide assessment, safety, support, and treatment referrals.[58] In Australia, there is a Crisis Assessment and Treatment Team that responds to a psychiatric crisis situation with trained mental health professionals.[59] SafetyNet is the system used in the Netherlands that provides case management and crisis response to individuals with complex mental health needs.[60] And Sweden uses the Psychiatric Emergency Response Team ambulance. A paramedic and two mental health nurses respond to psychiatric crisis intervention.[61]

Mental health is a spectrum that can range from mental wellness to severe mental illness. There are multiple types of community-based mental health treatment services that can be developed to assist in establishing environments that are conducive to meeting the mental health needs of its inhabitants. Plus, given the known fact that trauma impacts mental wellness, we should view well-established community mental health systems as a necessity. By promoting mental well-being and preventing trauma, communities could impact the mental health of many individuals in their populace.

BOX 7.1 A Critical Thinking Synopsis—Do You Agree?

Provision of well-established and effective community-based mental health services can be obtained in countries through organized efforts within each community and state. The meta-community and balanced care models both address the needed systems to sustain optimum mental health within a populace and should be used as guidance in the implementation of psychiatric services that can meet mental health recipients' needs.

In this chapter, data has been provided that substantiates the benefits of each aspect within community-based mental health care that are required to meet minimum standards of care.

Main Points

1. The balanced care model makes the case for both hospital and community-based mental health services to adequately meet the needs of those populations requiring psychiatric services.
2. Community mental health can be described as the principles and practices needed to promote mental health for a local population by
   a. addressing population needs in ways that are accessible and acceptable;
   b. building on the goals and strengths of people who experience mental illness;
   c. promoting a wide network of supports, services, and resources of adequate capacity; and
   d. emphasizing services that are both evidence-based and recovery oriented.
3. The meta-community model considers a broader range of services, such as social, housing and homelessness services, justice, education, and employment. Following this holistic approach, the analysis of the mental health balance of care should not be restricted to just the hospital and community care.
4. For community-based mental health systems to function effectively, each community must include the provision of each client's housing needs, as it is a basic need for recovery.
5. In 1997, the Robert Wood Johnson Foundation, the SAMSA, several State Departments of Mental Health, and additional private foundations initiated a national demonstration to implement six specific evidence-based practices that were deemed essential community mental health services, including systematic medication management, ACT, SE, family psychoeducation, IMR, and integrated treatment for co-occurring disorders.

6. ACT is a multidisciplinary team approach with assistive outreach in the community for individuals with severe mental illness who are at risk for psychiatric crisis, hospitalization, and involvement with the criminal justice system.
7. The Community Mental Health Services Block Grant program makes funds available to all 50 states. The funds can be used for new programs or to supplement existing programs.
8. Mobile crisis health teams are mental health professionals who respond to crises or emergency situations and assist in decreasing psychiatric hospitalizations, stabilizing the client, and decreasing imprisonment. It has been identified that the benefits of crisis teams include stabilization of mental health, improved safety, suicide prevention, family support, increased navigation with services, and cost-effectiveness.

Notes

1. Thornicroft, Graham et al. (2013), The balanced care model: The case for both hospital- and community-based mental healthcare, *Br J Psychiatry,* 102(4), https://pubmed.ncbi.nlm.nih.gov/23549938/ (accessed January 18, 2018), pp. 246–248.
2. Thornicroft, Graham et al. (2013), The balanced care model: The case for both hospital- and community-based mental healthcare, *Br J Psychiatry,* 102(4), https://pubmed.ncbi.nlm.nih.gov/23549938/ (accessed January 18, 2018), pp. 246–248.
3. Almeda, Nerea et al. (2022), Modeling the balance of care: Impact of an evidence-informed policy on a mental health ecosystem, *PlosOne,* 17(1): e0261621, https://www.ncbi.nlm.nih.gov/pmc/articles/PMC8752022/ (accessed August 23, 2023).
4. Thornicroft, Graham et al. (2016), Community mental health care worldwide: Current status and further developments, *World Psychiatry,* 15(3), https://pubmed.ncbi.nlm.nih.gov/27717265/ (accessed January 18, 2018), pp. 276–286.
5. Harvard Health Publishing (2014), *The homeless mentally ill,* Harvard Medical School, http://health.harvard.edu/newsletter_article/the_homeless_mentally_ill (accessed January 18, 2018).
6. Harvard Health Publishing (2014), *The homeless mentally ill,* Harvard Medical School, http://health.harvard.edu/newsletter_article/the_homeless_mentally_ill (accessed January 18, 2018).
7. HUD (2022), *HUD releases 2021 annual homeless assessment report, Part I,* https://www.hud.gov/press/press_releases_media_advisories/HUD_No_22_022 (accessed August 23, 2023).
8. Distasio, Jino (2017), *Homelessness costs Canadians big money without addressing the causes,* https://evidencenetwork.ca/homelessness-costs-canadians-big-money-without-addressing-the-causes/ (accessed August 23, 2023).
9. Crisis UK (2021), *Cost of homelessness,* https://www.crisis.org.uk/ending-homelessness/homelessness-knowledge-hub/cost-of-homelessness/ (accessed August 23, 2023).
10. McPherson, Peter et al. (2018), Mental health supported Accommodation Services: A systematic review of mental health and psychosocial outcomes, *BMC Psychiatry,* 18:12, https://doi.org/10.1186/s12888-018-1725-8 (accessed August 24, 2023).

11. Bouras, Nick et al. (2018), From community to meta-community mental health care, *Int J Environ Res Public Health*, 15(4), https://www.ncbi.nlm.nih.gov/pmc/articles/PMC5923848/ (accessed August 23, 2023), pp. 806.

12. Bouras, Nick et al. (2018), From community to meta-community mental health care, *Int J Environ Res Public Health*, 15(4), https://www.ncbi.nlm.nih.gov/pmc/articles/PMC5923848/ (accessed August 23, 2023), pp. 806.

13. Bouras, Nick et al. (2018), From community to meta-community mental health care, *Int J Environ Res Public Health*, 15(4), https://www.ncbi.nlm.nih.gov/pmc/articles/PMC5923848/ (accessed August 23, 2023), pp. 806.

14. Drake, Robert and Latimer, Eric. (2012). Lessons learned in developing community mental health in North America, *World Psychiatry*, 11(1), https://www.ncbi.nlm.nih.gov/pmc/articles/PMC3266763/ (accessed February 1, 2018), pp. 47–51.

15. Morant, Nicola, PhD et al. (2016), Shared decision making for psychiatric medication management: Beyond the micro-social, health expectations, *An International Journal of Public Participation in Health Care and Health Policy*, 19(5), https://pubmed.ncbi.nlm.nih.gov/26260361/ (accessed February 4, 2018), pp. 1002–1014.

16. Velligan, Dawn et al. (2017), *Why do psychiatric patients stop antipsychotic medications? A systemic review of reasons for non-adherence to medication in patients with serious mental illness*, Dove Press, 11, https://www.ncbi.nlm.nih.gov/pmc/articles/PMC5344423/#:~:text=This%20systematic%20review%20suggests%20that%20a%20negati ve%20attitude,reasons%20may%20improve%20adherence%20in%20a%20high-risk%20group (accessed February 4, 2018), pp. 449–468.

17. Deng M. et al. (2022), Factors influencing medication adherence among patients with severe mental disorders from the perspective of mental health professionals, *BMC Psychiatry*, 22(1), https://www.ncbi.nlm.nih.gov/pmc/articles/PMC8740063/ (accessed August 23, 2023), pp. 22.

18. Velligan, Dawn et al. (2017), *Why do psychiatric patients stop antipsychotic medications? A systemic review of reasons for non-adherence to medication in patients with serious mental illness*, Dove Press, 11, https://www.ncbi.nlm.nih.gov/pmc/articles/PMC5344423/#:~:text=This%20systematic%20review%20suggests%20that%20a%20negati ve%20attitude,reasons%20may%20improve%20adherence%20in%20a%20high-risk%20group (accessed February 4, 2018), pp. 449–468.

19. Sherman, Laura, PhD et al. (2017), Availability of supported employment in specialty mental health treatment facilities and facility characteristics: 2014, *The CBHSQ Report*, Substance Abuse and Mental Health Services Administration. https://pubmed.ncbi.nlm.nih.gov/28749638/ (accessed February 4, 2018), pp. 1–9.

20. Guhne, Uta et al. (2021), Employment status and desire to work in severe mental illness: results from an observational, cross-sectional study, *Soc Psychiatry Psychiatr Epidemiol*, 56(9), https://ww.ncbi.nlm.nih.gov/pmc/articles/PMC8429146/ (accessed August 23, 2023), pp.1657–1667.

21. U.S. Legal, *Supported employment laws and legal definition*, https://definitions.uslegal.com/s/supported-employment/ (accessed February 1, 2018).

22. Luciano, Alison, MPH and Meara, Ellen, PhD (2014), The employment status of people with mental illness: National survey data from 2009–2010, *Psychiatric Serv* 65(10), https://pubmed.ncbi.nlm.nih.gov/24933361/ (accessed February 4, 2018), pp. 1201–1209.

23. SAMHSA (2014), *Transforming lives through supported employment program*, https://samhsa.gov/criminal-juvilie-justice/grant-grantess/transforming-lives-through-supported-employment-program (accessed February 1, 2018).

24. Cooper, Stephanie (2022), *Division of mental health services greatly expands supported employment initiative across the state*, Tennessee Works, https://www.tennesseeworks.org/division-of-mental-health-services-greatly-expands-supported-employment-initiative-across-the- state/#:~:text=Data%20shows%20that%2066%25%20of%20individuals%20living%20with,have%20access%20to%20an%20evidence-based%20supported%20employment%20model (accessed August 23, 2023).

25. Park, A-La et al. (2022), Economic analyses of supported employment programmes for people with mental health conditions: A systematic review, *European Psychiatry*, 65(1), https://pubmed.ncbi.nlm.nih.gov/35983840/ (accessed August 24, 2023).

26. Srivastava, Prashant and Panday, Rishi (2017), Psychoeducation an Effective Tool as Treatment 2 Modality in Mental Health, *The International Journal of Indian Psychology*, 4(1), 82. https://ijip.in/articles/psychoeducation-an-effective-tool-as-treatment-modality-in-mental-health/#:~:text=Psychoeducation%20is%20understood%20as%20systematic%2C%20structured%2C%20didactic%20information,effective%20tool%20as%20treatment%20modality%20in%20mental%20Health (accessed March 4, 2018), pp. 123–130.

27. Zhoa, Sai, Sampson et al. (2015), *Psychoeducation (brief) for people with serious mental illness*, Cochrane Database of Systematic Reviews, Issue 4, ART, https://www.academia.edu/21897562/Psychoeducation_brief_for_people_with_serious_mental_illness (accessed March 4, 2918), pp.1.

28. Nash, Jo, PhD (2021), *How to perform psychoeducation interventions: 14 topics*, https://positivepsychology.com/psychoeducation/#google_vignette (accessed August 23, 2023).

29. Sujit, Sarkhel et al. (2020), Clinical practice guidelines for psychoeducation in psychiatric disorders general principles of psychoeducation, *Indian J Psychiatry*, Supp 2, https://www.ncbi.nlm.nih.gov/pmc/articles/PMC7001357/ (accessed August 23, 2023), pp. 319–323.

30. Harvy, Carol (2018), *Family psychoeducation for people living with schizophrenia and their families*, Cambridge University Press, https://www.cambridge.org/core/journals/bjpsych-advances/article/family-psychoeducation-for-people-living-with-schizophrenia-and-their-families/1F624040803C69204CB936C7826185E3 (accessed August 24, 2023).

31. Substance Abuse and Mental Health Services Administration (2009), *Illness and management recovery*, U.S. Department of Health and Human Services, No. SMA-09-4462, https://store.samhsa.gov/sites/default/files/d7/priv/practitionerguidesandhandouts_0.pdf (accessed March 8, 2018), pp. 2

32. Substance Abuse and Mental Health Services Administration (2009), *Illness and management recovery*, U.S. Department of Health and Human Services, No. SMA-09-4462, https://store.samhsa.gov/sites/default/files/d7/priv/practitionerguidesandhandouts_0.pdf (accessed March 8, 2018), pp. 24.

33. Substance Abuse and Mental Health Services Administration (2009), *Illness and management recovery*, U.S. Department of Health and Human Services, No. SMA-09-4462, https://store.samhsa.gov/sites/default/files/d7/priv/practitionerguidesandhandouts_0.pdf (accessed March 8, 2018), pp. 252.

34. Devendorf, Andrew et al. (2022), Optimal well-being after psychopathology: Prevalence and correlates, *Clinical Psychological Science*, https://doi.org/10.1177/21677026221078872 (accessed May 13, 2022).

35. Devendorf, Andrew et al. (2022), Optimal well-being after psychopathology: Prevalence and correlates, *Clinical Psychological Science*, https://doi.org/10.1177/21677026221078872 (accessed May 13, 2022).

36. Roosenschoon Bert-Jan et al. (2021), Effects of illness management and recovery: A multi-center randomized controlled trial, *Front Psychiatry*, 14, 12:723435, https://www.ncbi.nlm.nih.gov/pmc/articles/PMC8712643/ (accessed August 23, 2023).

37. Roosenschoon Bert-Jan et al. (2021), Effects of illness management and recovery: A multi-center randomized controlled trial, *Front Psychiatry*, 14, 12:723435, https://www.ncbi.nlm.nih.gov/pmc/articles/PMC8712643/ (accessed August 23, 2023).

38. Substance Abuse and Mental Health Services Administration (2009), *Integrated treatment for co-occurring disorders*, U.S. Department of Health and Human Services, No. SMA-08-4366, https://store.samhsa.gov/sites/default/files/d7/priv/ebp-kit-the-evidence-10242019.pdf (accessed March 8, 2018), pp. 4.

39. Kelly, Thomas and Daley, Dennis (2013), Integrated treatment of substance use and psychiatric disorders, *Soc Work Public Health*, 28(0), https://pubmed.ncbi.nlm.nih.gov/23731427/ (accessed March 8, 2018), pp. 388–406.

40. McClean Hospital (2020), *Dual diagnosis: Barriers and gateways to effective addiction care*, https://www.mcleanhospital.org/essential/dual-diagnosis-barriers-and-gateways-effective-addiction-care (accessed August 24, 2023).

41. Ford II, James et al. (2021), Improving medication access within integrated treatment for individuals with co-occurring disorders in substance use treatment agencies, *Sage Journals*, https://doi.org/10.1177/26334895211033659 (accessed October 26, 2021).

42. Healthy Connections Medicaid (2023), *Addition of assertive community treatment services*, https://www.scdhhs.gov/communications/addition-assertive-community-treatment-services#:~:text=Effective%20July%201%2C%202023%2C%20the%20South%20Carolina%20Department,2023%2C%20to%20reflect%20the%20addition%20of%20these%20services (accessed August 24, 2023).

43. SAMHSA (2023), *Certified community behavioral health centers*, https://www.samhsa.gov/certified-community-behavioral-health-clinics (accessed August 23, 2023).

44. National Alliance on Mental Illness (2023), *Certified community behavioral health clinics*, https://www.nami.org/Advocacy/Policy-Priorities/Improving-Health/Certified-Community-Behavioral-Health-Clinics#:~:text=Specifically%2C%20CCBHCs%20must%20provide%3A%201%2024%2F7%20mobile%20crisis,services%208%20Peer%20and%20family%20supports%20More%20items (accessed August 24, 2023).

45. Definitive Healthcare (2023), *How many federally qualified health centers are there?* https://www.definitivehc.com/blog/how-many-fqhcs-are-there (accessed August 25, 2023).

46. Department of Health and Human Services (2021), *SAMSHA awards record-setting $825 million in grants to strengthen community mental health centers, and support Americans living with serious emotional disturbances, mental illnesses*, https://www.hhs.gov/about/news/2021/09/28/samsha-awards-record-setting-825-million-in-grants-strengthen-Community (accessed October 30, 2021).

47. Association for Community Mental Health Centers (2021), *Why is funding for community mental health centers (CMHCs) important*, https://www.acmhck.org/resources/why-is-funding-for-comunity-mental-health-centers-important (accessed October 30, 2021).

48. World Health Organization (2021), *New WHO guidance seeks to put an end to human rights violations in mental health care*, https://www.who.int/news/item/10-06-2021-new-whos-guidance-seeks-to-put-an-end-to-human-rights-violations-in-mental-health-care (accessed October 30, 2021).

49. Substance Abuse and Mental Health Services Administration (2021), *National mental health services survey (N-MHSS): 2020 data on mental health treatment facilities*, Center for Behavioral Health Statistics and Quality. https://www.samhsa.gov/data/report/national-mental-health-services-survey-n-mhss-2020-data-mental-health-treatment-facilities (accessed April 6, 2022), pp. 22.

50. Unicef (2021), *Community-based mental health care in Peru*, https://www.unicef.org/stories/community-based-mental-health-care-in-peru (accessed May 9, 2022).

51. Wong Hoi-Ching, Ben et al. (2022), Transitioning to community-based mental healthcare: Reform experiences of five countries, *BiPsych International*, 19(1), https://www.cambridge.org/core/journals/bjpsych-international/article/transitioning-to-communitybased-mental-healthcare-reform-experiences-of-five-countries/35A94E06F0ABCD79515AFB3B-46FAE9FC (accessed January 4, 2023), pp. 18–21.

52. Wong Hoi-Ching, Ben et al. (2022), Transitioning to community-based mental healthcare: Reform experiences of five countries, *BiPsych International*, 19(1), https://www.cambridge.org/core/journals/bjpsych-international/article/transitioning-to-communitybased-mental-healthcare-reform-experiences-of-five-countries/35A94E06F0ABCD79515AFB3B-46FAE9FC (accessed January 4, 2023), pp. 18–21.

53. Carmona, Jaime et al. (2021), *Community mental health care in Mexico: A regional perspective from a mid-income country, International Journal of Mental Health Systems*, 15, Article 7, https://doi.org/10.1186/s130330929099429-9 (accessed May 9, 2022).

54. International Mental Health Collaborating Network (2022), *24-7 community mental health centres*, https://www.imhcn.org/bibliography/recent-innovations-and-good-practices/community-mental-health-centres (accessed May 9, 2022).

55. National Alliance on Mental Illness (2022), *Crisis response*, https://www.nami.org/advocacy/policy-priorities/responding-to-crisis/crisis-response (accessed May 8, 2022).

56. National Alliance on Mental Illness (2022), *Crisis intervention team (CIT) programs*, https://www.nami.org/advocacy/crisis-intervention/crisis-intervention-team-programs (accessed May 8, 2022).

57. U.S. Department of Health and Human Services (2022), *HHS announces more than $100 million in bipartisan safer communities act funds for states and territories to improve mental health services*, https://www.hhs.gov/about/news/2022/10/21/hhs-announces-more-100-million-bipartisan-safer-communities-act-funds-states-territories-improve-mental-health-services.html#:~:text=SAMHSA%20recommended%20that%20states%20and%20territories%20use%20the,call%20centers%2C%20child%20welfare%20organizations%2C%20schools%20and%20others (accessed August 24, 2023).

58. SAMHSA (2023), 988 Lifeline Performance Metrics, https://www.samhsa.gov/find-help/988/performance-metrics,(accessed August 23, 2023).

59. Treatment Advocacy Center (2019), *Research weekly: Beyond road runners: Insights from other countries*, https://www.treatmentadvocacycenter.org/fixing-the-system/features-and-news/4168-research-weekly-beyond-road-runners (accessed May 9, 2022).

60. Treatment Advocacy Center (2019), *Research weekly: Beyond road runners: Insights from other countries*, https://www.treatmentadvocacycenter.org/fixing-the-system/features-and-news/4168-research-weekly-beyond-road-runners (accessed May 9, 2022).

61. Treatment Advocacy Center (2019), *Research weekly: Beyond road runners: Insights from other countries*, https://www.treatmentadvocacycenter.org/fixing-the-system/features-and-news/4168-research-weekly-beyond-road-runners (accessed May 9, 2022).

Credits

Fig. 7.1: Data Source: Alison Luciano and Ellen Meara, "Employment Status of People With Mental Illness: National Survey Data From 2009 and 2010," Psychiatric Services, vol. 65, no. 10, 2014.

Fig. 7.2: Data Source: Andrew R. Devendorf, Ruba Rum, Todd B. Kashdan, and Jonathan Rottenberg, "Optimal Well-Being After Psychopathology: Prevalence and Correlates," Clinical Psychological Science, vol. 10, no. 5, 2022.

Fig. 7.3: Data Source: https://www.datafiles.samhsa.gov/dataset/national-mental-health-services-survey-2020-n-mhss-2020-ds0001

Fig. 7.4: Source: https://www.hhs.gov/about/news/2022/10/21/hhs-announces-more-100-million-bipartisan-safer-communities-act-funds-states-territories-improve-mental-health-services.html#:~:text=SAMHSA%20recommended%20that%20states%20and%20territories%20use%20the,call%20cent.

CHAPTER 8

Primary Care Providers, Telemental Health, Hospital-Based Psychiatric Units, and Governmental Strategies

The main objective of this chapter is for the reader to comprehend that primary care providers, telemental health, hospital-based psychiatric units, and governmental strategies are essential components of effective community mental healthcare systems.

In this chapter, additional strategies/systems to improve access to mental health services are presented to establish further comprehension of the global mental healthcare crisis and ways to promote quality of life. These systems include hospital-based inpatient treatment, primary care providers, telemental health, trauma-informed care, day hospitals, child and adolescent units, crisis centers, and governmental strategies. Each component is an important aspect in meeting clients' psychiatric treatment requirements to obtain recovery and sustain stability within community-based mental health care.

Hospital Treatment Facilities

Public mental health facilities, private free-standing psychiatric hospitals, and psychiatric units in general hospitals are the most common types of inpatient treatment settings. Public psychiatric facilities are operated by state or county governments. Free-standing private mental health hospitals are operated by nonprofit or for-profit corporations. And psychiatric units in general hospitals can be operated by government, nonprofit, or for-profit entities.

United States

When the Medicaid program was established in 1965, Congress underscored that the costs for state and local psychiatric hospitals should not be funded by this resource. The Institution for Mental Disease (IMD) exclusion rule was implemented; this rule continues to exclude state psychiatric hospitals and any hospital in which more than 50% of the beds are occupied by clients with a primary mental health diagnosis from reimbursement for care provided to Medicaid beneficiaries between the ages of 21 and 64.[1] Because of federal reimbursement standards and regulatory structures, state psychiatric hospitals have depended predominately on state funding.

Rules and regulations governing psychiatric units and hospitals are described in each states Health and Human Services Licensing Requirements. It is broadly accepted that the licensing regulations were formulated and implemented to protect the health, safety, and welfare of clients and employees in psychiatric hospitals/units.

Behavioral Health Units

General hospitals began implementing psychiatric/behavioral health units (BHUs) into their specialty fields in the late 1940s to early 1950s. By 1960, there were more than 600 psychiatric units located in general hospital settings within the nation. This process was approached more earnestly in the late 1970s, developing small inpatient psychiatric units in general hospitals that were not IMDs; thus, the utilization of general hospitals grew as an alternative to state psychiatric hospitals in the United States. But, in some regions, BHUs are still not in existence.

In 2021, protestors marched in Bozeman, Montana, to address the lack of inpatient care for people with mental health issues at Bozeman Health Deaconess Hospital. Colette Kirchhoff, a family practice and hospice physician, stated, "We need inpatient psychiatric care beds when someone is having a (crisis), they need to be able to stay in our town."[2]

Bozeman resident and actor Glenn Close held a sign that read "Mental Health Empowers," stating, "For me, it is a family thing, the stigma is so huge, but it's just part of being a human being."[3]

Today, modern hospital settings include BHUs that are used for short-term stays inside general hospitals. These units are used for the stabilization of acute psychiatric episodes. Focusing on providing a safe, secure environment where individuals experiencing crisis can receive therapeutic care, BHUs are locked treatment areas that provide lower environmental stress levels, open and communal spaces, and limit visitation to facilitate recovery. A multidisciplinary team is provided that includes nurses, psychiatrists, therapists, psychologists, social workers, and behavioral technicians. There are multiple treatment modalities offered on these units:

1. Medication stabilization
2. Individual, group, music, and art therapy
3. Physical and occupational therapy
4. Coordination of community resources
5. Electroconvulsive therapy
6. Education

Psychiatric Hospital or Unit Licensing Requirements

Initial licenses for a psychiatric-based treatment entity are issued when the state licensing division receives a completed application with appropriate monetary fees, and the institution meets all the state-mandated requirements for the operation of a psychiatric/behavioral unit or psychiatric hospital. Annual renewal and initial issuance of a license will be considered by the state licensing division, with weight being placed on the Health and Human Services Survey deficiencies, Life Safety Code deficiencies, complaint investigations and resolutions, compliance with laws and standards surrounding communicable and reportable diseases, and the institutional implementation and effectiveness of quality assurance management programs within a specific psychiatric unit or hospital.[4]

The current license shall be placed in a public area for all to view within a psychiatric institution or unit. And each state's regulations mandate that every psychiatric institution shall develop and maintain a governing body that is legally responsible for the management and operations of the unit or hospital, including the implementation of bylaws that depict each governing member's responsibilities.

Physical Environment

Construction or development of the physical environment in a mental health unit or hospital shall encompass regions for private conversations, therapy sessions, group activities, dining, and recreational programs. Every psychiatric facility will have sufficient space to accommodate the number of clients they will serve. A minimum of one detention room will be implemented within each psychiatric unit/hospital.[5] And Life Safety Code requirements will be met within each facility to maintain client, staff, and visitor safety.

A medical library shall be available to all medical and nursing staff that contains resources that are current and applicable to modern services provided within each psychiatric unit/hospital. Facilities shall either provide on-campus or contract out to other entities services of laboratory testing, radiology, and pharmaceutical supplies. Housekeeping, laundry, and maintenance services will be provided within each hospital or unit to sustain a safe and sanitary living environment for all clients served in a psychiatric setting.

There are several studies that have been conducted that demonstrate that a psychiatric unit's physical environment can be directly correlated to the levels and episodes of aggression demonstrated by clients. Some of these studies have demonstrated the impact of physical design on emotional states, behavior, and patient outcomes. Variables included in the studies were types of rooms, the amount of private and public space, natural lighting, views, atmosphere, and safety measures. Most of the studies concluded that the intervention factor of seclusion to manage aggressive clients was significantly higher in forensic units versus admission or nonadmission units.[6]

Also, client exposure to natural elements, such as gardens, plants, and landscape paintings, has demonstrated positive effects, including comfort, psychological well-being, decreased fatigue, and stress, resulting in lower behavioral incidents. The amount of client private space had a significant impact on behavioral outbursts because of feelings of territorial control, feelings of ownership, identity, a sense of dignity, and regulation of social interaction. Lack of comfort and personal control over the physical environment can be a contributing factor that leads to distress and helplessness for psychiatric clients.[7] Even today, problems still exist in some state psychiatric hospitals, as portrayed in Box 8.1.

BOX 8.1 Montana State Hospital

In April of 2022, the Montana State Psychiatric Hospital was decertified by the Federal Centers for Medicare and Medicaid Services; the facility failed to meet Medicare's basic health and safety requirements. And there had been eight substantiated abuse and neglect reports.

State health department director Charlie Brereton stated, "We've stabilized MSH since the decertification with a change in leadership and with no significant increase in deaths, serious injuries, or substantiated abuse or neglect allegations."[8]

Psychiatric Services

Inpatient psychiatric services should be part of an overall plan of care, supporting a coordinated effort between the patient, family, treatment team, and outpatient service providers. Facilities that provide mental health services shall maintain a chief psychiatrist on staff who possesses a doctoral degree in psychology.[9] The lead psychiatrist will ensure that adequate staffing is maintained to meet each client's requirements, encompassing evaluations, diagnosis, program development, research, and therapeutic interventions.

Each psychiatric client, upon admission to a mental health institution, must have a provisional or admitting psychiatric diagnosis and comorbid diseases (if applicable) diagnosis at the time of admission. A psychiatric evaluation must be completed on each client within 60 hours of admission, which includes a medical history.[10] Clients can be admitted both on a voluntary or involuntary basis; if a patient poses an immediate safety risk to themselves or others because of symptoms of mental illness, they can be admitted to a psychiatric unit against their will.

Staffing

All inpatient psychiatric treatment facilities should be staffed with sufficient numbers of qualified professional, technical, and consultation personnel to sufficiently formulate, implement, and evaluate a comprehensive treatment program for each psychiatric patient.

Nursing services shall be conducted under the supervision of a registered nurse, such as the director of nursing. A director of nursing will direct, monitor, and evaluate the nursing services provided in a psychiatric hospital/unit. Facilities will maintain adequate numbers of professional staff to meet patient population needs. Figure 8.1 illustrates the turnover percentage rates of employees in state and nonstate inpatient mental health treatment facilities in Texas.

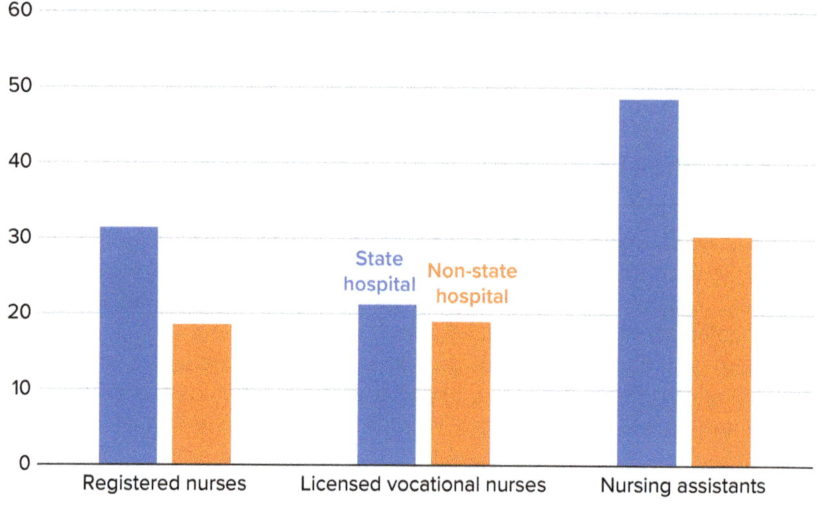

FIGURE 8.1 Employee Turnover Rates.[12]

An analysis in 2022 of staff turnover rates at behavioral health facilities revealed the rate averaging around 31.3%. Across seven job classifications, turnover rates ranged from an average of 17.37% for supervisors to 37.17% for mental health workers/psychiatric aides. The turnover rates by job classification were as follows: supervisors: 17.37%, clinical professionals: 22.91%, top-level executives: 24.61%, licensed practical nurses: 26.43%, registered nurses: 29.36%, and mental health workers/psychiatric aides: 37.17%.[11]

Each facility shall maintain a medical or clinical director on staff who is qualified to provide leadership with psychiatric services. Physicians and psychiatrists shall be adequate in number to meet the requirements of each institution's patient population.

Individualized Treatments

As discussed previously, every psychiatric client will have a developed and implemented comprehensive treatment plan that addresses strengths and disabilities, including the following:

- A substantiated diagnosis
- Short-term and long-term goals
- Specific treatment modalities used
- Responsibilities of each member of the treatment team
- Adequate documentation to verify the diagnosis and treatment modalities[13]

The treatment plan will provide clear goals and measurable outcomes and must address the specific actions that triggered a psychiatric crisis. The care plan should be in a format that is meaningful to the client and in language that is easy for the patient to understand. There should be clearly identified timescales for review and evidence that the process is occurring, adjusting the treatment plan as necessary to obtain effective outcomes. Social, recreational, spiritual, treatment, and community needs should be identified in the care plan to provide a holistic approach to the care plan process. The formulated plan of treatment will be expected to improve the client's condition and/or assist in the formulation of a substantiating diagnosis.

Other Countries

BHUs in general hospitals have been implemented all over the world. According to WHO and Our World in Data, from 2017 to 2019, the countries with the most BHUs were Argentina, Belize, Ghana, Hungary, Iceland, Monaco, Australia, Spain, and Saint Kitts and Nevis.[14,15]

Regulatory guidelines for BHUs vary across countries. A comparison of mental health legislation in five developed countries (the Republic of Ireland, England and Wales, Scotland, Ontario, Canada), and Victoria (Australia) was conducted to describe similarities and differences in mental health legislation between the jurisdictions. The study found that across the five jurisdictions examined, largely similar procedures for admission, detention, and treatment of involuntary patients are employed, reflecting adherence to international standards and incorporation of human rights-based principles. Differences existed in relation to the criteria to define a mental disorder, the occurrence of automatic review hearings in a timely fashion after a patient is involuntarily admitted, and the role of supported decision-making under mental health legislation.[16] In addition, there are acute day hospitals and crisis houses.

Day Hospitals and Crisis Houses

Day hospital treatment is typically used in cases where continuous inpatient treatment is not required, for follow-up after an inpatient stay, as an extension of outpatient treatment, and for rehabilitation. These treatment facilities decrease the gap between outpatient care and full inpatient hospital admission and have been implemented in many countries.

Crisis houses also exist in some countries and provide short-term, intensive support to manage acute psychiatric episodes in a residential setting. Some will accept self-referrals, while others require a mental health practitioner's referral. It has been argued by some advocates that these facilities could potentially assist in de-stigmatizing the option of inpatient psychiatric treatment. There is variance in the stay length with these facilities, from several nights to four weeks. Typical services focus on defining and limiting the crisis, planning for the immediate and long-term future, and securing appropriate community, family, and personal resources. Children and adolescents who experience mental health decline or conditions may require additional assistance, and specialized units have been developed for this purpose.

Child and Adolescent Units

In 1972, individuals under the age of 21 were exempted from the IMD exclusion, which led to the increase of free-standing psychiatric hospitals operating child and adolescent units.[17] Scientists who work searching for causes of mental illness study the development of the brain from birth to adulthood. This research has revealed that maturation of the human brain does not occur until the early 20s and that the teenage brain goes through several changes during adolescence. Genetics, childhood experiences, and the environment in which an individual resides when reaching adolescence will all shape their adult behavior.

Child and adolescent psychiatric inpatient units offer comprehensive diagnostic evaluation and treatment to individuals, typically from the ages of 5 to 17, with emotional and behavioral problems, including anxiety disorders, psychotic disorders, mood disorders, severe disruptive behaviors, and suicidal thoughts and attempts. Children must exhibit the following:

- A serious functional impairment
- At risk of disruption of a preferred living or childcare environment due to psychiatric symptoms
- Enrolled in a school system's special education program because of serious emotional disturbance[18]

Treatment programs and plans generally include a combination of psychotherapy, behavior management, family counseling, and pharmacological management. Staff will provide interventions designed to relieve acute psychiatric symptomatology and restore the child/adolescent's ability to function in a less restrictive environment.

It is estimated that more than 7% of adolescents 13 to 17 years of age have been diagnosed with anxiety, and more than 36% of children with behavioral problems have been diagnosed with anxiety disorders.[19] When anxiety becomes an excessive, irrational dread of everyday situations, it becomes a disabling condition that can include obsessive-compulsive disorder, post-traumatic stress disorder, social phobia, specific phobia, and generalized anxiety disorder. Symptoms of many of these conditions begin in childhood or adolescence. Brain imaging, molecular biology, and genetic mapping research are revealing brain mechanisms involved in anxiety disorders that have the potential to lead to earlier identification and better treatment modalities.

According to WHO, depression is estimated to occur among 1.1% of adolescents aged 10–14 years and 2.8% of 15- to 19-year-olds.[20] Children who are depressed may exhibit different symptomatology than adults, such as complaining of feeling sick, refusing to go to school, clinging to parents or a caregiver, or they may worry excessively that a parent may die. Adolescents who are depressed may sulk, get into trouble at school, be negative or grouchy, or feel misunderstood. It is being suggested by many professionals that primary care needs to become more involved in mental health care, especially in lower income countries.

Mental Health Services Integrated Into Primary Care Settings

Remember, there is overwhelming evidence that there is a definitive connection between mental and physical health, and this understanding supports the integration of mental health services into the primary care setting. Several supportive factors for this process are (1) it could assist in decreasing stigma and discrimination associated with mental illness; (2) there is a potential for improvement in the overall health of individuals; (3) it supports continuity of care; (4) it is an affordable avenue for providing mental health services; (5) it provides easy accessibility to services for individuals experiencing mental conditions.

In communities where challenges are apparent for the delivery of mental health services, there is a growing need for general practitioner involvement to meet the needs of individuals experiencing mental illness. Many individuals with poor mental health can be diagnosed and treated in the primary care setting. It is strongly recommended that healthcare providers should educate themselves on screening recommendations, behavioral health, trauma-informed care, telepsychiatry, and mental health disparities. The American Academy of Family Physicians recommends screening all adult clients for depression with routine health visits. Early identification of depression can enhance recovery, prevent relapse, and decrease emotional and economic burdens.

A more holistic approach to well-being and health is developed by incorporating mental health care into primary care settings through a collaboration of mental healthcare providers and integrating primary and preventative medicine into mental/behavioral healthcare services. The traditional mental healthcare system should merge with primary care to develop comprehensive healthcare delivery systems.

The collaborative care model is an evidence-based approach for integrating physical and behavioral health services within the primary care–based Medicaid health home model, among other settings.[21] The basic elements of the model are a primary care provider-led team driven to deliver care coordination and management, regular monitoring, and psychiatric caseload reviews and consultation. Long-term analyses have demonstrated that $1 spent on collaborative care saves $6.50 in health care costs.[22] The Health Home State Plan Option is for people with Medicaid who have two or more chronic conditions, have one chronic condition and are at risk for a second, and/or have one serious and persistent mental health condition. There is also increased discussion of providing trauma-informed care across all healthcare settings.

Trauma-Informed Care

Trauma-informed care is a delivery of services that promotes recovery and healing from trauma rather than practices that retraumatize individuals. It has been established that exposure to trauma predisposes individuals to poor physical and mental health. There are several guiding principles of trauma-informed care, including safety, trust, choice, peer support, collaboration, cultural/gender issues, and empowerment. It is estimated that at least 70% (223.4 million people) of adults have experienced some type of traumatic event at least once in their lives.[23]

The American Medical Association has adopted a policy of trauma-informed care that recognizes the widespread impact of trauma on patients, identifies the signs and symptoms of trauma, and treats patients by fully integrating knowledge about trauma into procedures to avoid retraumatization.[24] Universal trauma-informed care is gaining support, and best practices are evolving because of accumulative evidence of its benefits. Universal trauma precautions encompass treating all patients and families as if trauma is possible and implementing universal trauma-focused screening protocols. The California Academy of Family Physicians in 2020 launched the peer-to-peer learning workshops *Family Medicine Initiative on Trauma-Informed Care* to assist in improving family practice protocols with regard to trauma.[25] Primary care increased technology utilization during the COVID-19 pandemic; as a matter of fact, all branches of healthcare have now increased technological utilization to provide care in the industry.

Technology and Mental Health Treatment

Technology utilization in mental health treatment (e-mental health) ranges from support services, data collection, monitoring progress, tracking behaviors, and understanding mental well-being. Benefits related to e-mental health include being easily accessible, filling service gaps, saving the practitioner's time, providing flexibility, and being cost-effective. There are many avenues in technology that can be implemented for mental health, including telemental health (previously discussed), artificial intelligence, various mobile apps, and virtual reality. NIMH was awarded 404 grants, totaling $445 million, to study computer-based interventions designed to prevent or treat mental health conditions.

Virtual Reality

Virtual reality is being used in post-traumatic stress disorder, depression, anxiety, and other disorders. Mental health and wellness apps can be used that assist with mood, stress, and anxiety. There is variance with the mobile apps: some provide community-based support, others provide coaching and therapy sessions with trained professionals, others do self-management, and yet some assist with recovery and maintenance.

Artificial Intelligence

Artificial intelligence, such as Woebot and Wysa, is being implemented into mental health care. Woebot is an automated conversational agent designed to deliver cognitive behavioral therapy (CBT) in the format of brief daily conversations and mood tracking. Wysa is an emotionally intelligent chatbot that helps to manage thoughts and emotions via dialectical behavior therapy, guided meditation, and CBT. A 2021 published study on the utilization of chatbots revealed that the majority of respondents agreed that there are benefits associated with their utilization, such as that clients may disclose more information and that chatbots could increase activity or exercise, improve nutrition or diet, and improve medication and treatment adherence.[26]

eMEN Project

The eMEN project in Europe is developing applications for mental health prevention, diagnostics, and treatment to institute a blended care model where face-to-face and online treatment are combined. The partnering countries are Germany, the United Kingdom, the Netherlands, Belgium, Ireland, and France. The goal of the project is to increase e-mental health utilization to 15% by the end of the project, to at least 15% more five years after the project finishes, and to 60% ten years after the project finishes.[27]

TeleMental Health

Telehealth and telemental health, as we stated earlier, exploded with utilization during the COVID-19 pandemic. As the need for providing virtual mental health care services has increased, providers are finding ways to use phone and videoconferencing technology to bring therapy, evaluations, interventions, and medication management to clients. There are many positive attributes for the utilization of telemental health:

- Telemental health appointments provide more flexibility in scheduling appointments.
- The technology is available to a broader population of people, such as in remote areas.
- Telemental health services might be an easier first step for individuals.

The American Psychiatric Association (APA), in conjunction with the American Telemedicine Association (ATA), has released *Best Practices in Videoconferencing-Based Telemental Health*, a guide for providers who use telemental health, including telepsychiatry. The guide was co-written by the APA Committee on Telepsychiatry and the ATA Telemental Health Special Interest Group (TMH SIG). It is a consolidated update of previously published APA and ATA resources in telemental health and provides an overview of the use of clinical videoconferencing as a treatment medium.[28]

An analysis of telemental health utilization encompassed 196 articles, of the articles that specified a country, most mentioned the United States (31/196; 15.82%), followed by Italy and the United Kingdom, each with six articles (6/196; 3.06%). Using WHO's regions, most articles focused on the Americas (38/196; 19.39%) and Europe (32/196; 16.32%), followed by the Western Pacific (12/196; 6.12%), Southeast Asia (5/196; 2.55%), and the Eastern Mediterranean (3/196; 1.53%) and revealed that there was a marked growth in the uptake of telemental health during the pandemic and that telemental health is effective, safe, and will remain in use for the foreseeable future. Telemental health education should be incorporated into health professions curricula globally. With rapidly advancing technology and increasing acceptance of interactive online platforms among patients and healthcare providers, telemental health can provide sustainable mental healthcare across patient populations.[29] A few countries' governments have addressed telehealth and telemental health in their strategies for the improvement of mental healthcare systems.

Governmental Strategies to Improve Mental Health Services

Governments across the globe have recognized that the COVID-19 pandemic exposed and exacerbated the already broken mental healthcare delivery systems that exist in the majority of countries. There have been numerous legislative and policy changes worldwide in an attempt to address the mental healthcare crisis; we will briefly discuss a few of the implemented strategies in this section.

United States

In March of 2022, the Biden Administration released the "Fact Sheet: President Biden to Announce Strategy to Address Our National Mental Health Crisis, as Part of Unity Agenda in His First State of the Union." President Biden is laying out a vision to transform how mental health is understood, perceived, accessed, treated, and integrated—in and out of health care settings. "We cannot transform mental health solely through the health care system. We must also address the determinants of behavioral health, invest in community services, and foster a culture and environment that broadly promotes mental wellness and recovery. This crisis is not a medical one, but a societal one."[30] Some of the strategies presented include the following: The president's fiscal year (FY) 23 budget will invest $700 million in programs—like the National Health Service Corps, Behavioral Health Workforce Education and Training Program, and the Minority Fellowship Program—that provide training, access to scholarships, and loan repayment to mental health and SUD clinicians committed to practicing in rural and other underserved communities.[31]

In the fall of 2022, Health and Human Services (HHS) was expected to award over $225 million in training programs to increase the number of community health workers and other health support workers providing services, including behavioral health support, in underserved communities. The president's FY23 budget also proposed major new multiyear funding to develop provider capacity and support mental health transformation.[32] Additionally, there are state governors addressing the mental healthcare crisis. New York governor Kathy Hochul stated,

> Today marks a reversal in our state's approach to mental health care. This is a monumental shift to make sure no one falls through the cracks. The most significant change since the deinstitutionalization era of the 1970s. I'm proud to announce we will be investing more than $1 billion dollars and making critical policy changes to finally and fully meet the mental health needs of our state.[33]

The president's FY23 budget will build on granting states funding to expand CCBHCs for the communities that need them most. The president's budget will also permanently extend funding for CMHCs, which provide essential mental health services to vulnerable communities that would otherwise lack access.[34] Nevada governor Joe Lombardo is addressing community behavioral health centers to improve access to mental health care.

> My budget includes an enhancement in Medicaid to expand community behavioral health centers. This $17 million dollar expansion will add up to six clinics across the state in underserved areas including northern and rural Nevada. Ensuring more mental health services are available to anyone in need, regardless of their ability to pay.[35]

Plus, telemental health services have proven to be both safe and effective while reducing barriers to care. To maintain continuity of access, the administration will work with Congress to ensure coverage of telebehavioral health across health plans and support appropriate delivery of telemedicine across state lines. At the same time, the HHS will create a learning collaborative with state insurance departments to identify and address state-based barriers, like telehealth limitations, to behavioral health access.[36]

May of 2023

In May of 2023, the Biden-Harris administration announced new actions to tackle the nation's mental health crisis. They included critical actions to advance mental health improvement strategies across three key objectives: strengthening the mental health workforce and system capacity, connecting more Americans to care, and creating a continuum of support.[37] Some of the avenues for improvement included the following:

Through the Bipartisan Safer Communities Act, the Department of Education (ED) has awarded more than $280 million in funding to bolster the pipeline of mental health professionals serving in schools and expand school-based mental health services and supports. Earlier this week, ED announced that $95 million of this total was awarded in grants across 35 states to increase access to school-based mental health services and strengthen the pipeline of mental health professionals in high-needs school districts.[38] Arizona governor Katie Hobbs agrees that more work needs to be accomplished through the school systems:

> We need to prioritize hiring social workers and counselors for our schools to address the mental health crisis among children and teens. Currently each counselor in an Arizona school provides services for more than 700 kids on average. That's the highest ratio in the nation and nearly three times the recommended standard. That's unacceptable and we must do better.[39]

To ensure those in crisis have access to services, SAMHSA announced the availability of more than $200 million for states, territories, call centers, and tribal organizations to continue strengthening 988 operations.[40] It is simply too hard to know where to start when you or a loved one experiences a mental health challenge. That's why HHS launched FindSupport.Gov, a brand-new, easy-to-access, free-of-charge, and user-friendly online resource for all Americans to learn how to get support for mental health, drug, and alcohol issues.[41]

SAMHSA will award $6 million in suicide prevention grants across multiple programs to support states and tribes with implementing youth suicide prevention and early intervention strategies in schools, institutions of higher education, juvenile justice systems, substance use and mental health programs, foster care systems, and other child- and youth-serving organizations.[42]

SAMHSA will announce $5.4 million in grant awards for building communities of recovery to support the mobilization and connection of community-based resources to increase access to and quality of long-term recovery support for people with SUDs and co-occurring substance use and mental health disorders.[43] Governor Janet Mills of Maine and Governor Phil Scott of Vermont are both addressing substance misuse within their states:

> Governor Janet Mills: "As part of this budget, I am also proposing an historic $237 million in combined State and Federal funding for substance use disorder and mental health services, to include an increase in rates paid to providers. This will allow, for example, a 48% increase for methadone treatment and an 8.2% increase for intensive outpatient services, to complement an increase in recovery residences and a 24/7 drop-in center."[44]
>
> Governor Phil Scott: "Together, we made the state's largest-ever investment in substance abuse prevention, which is being deployed as we speak. It's helping community partners give students meaningful things to

do—like afterschool programs, clubs, sports and jobs – where they build healthy relationships, explore opportunities and feel valued."[45]

Canada

The Government of Canada announced in February of 2023 an investment of $196.1 billion over 10 years, including $46.2 billion in new funding, for provinces and territories to improve health care services for Canadians. This funding will be distributed partly through the Canada Health Transfer and partly through tailor-made bilateral agreements with provinces and territories that allow for flexibility for jurisdictional health care system needs. In addition, it will invest $2.5 billion over 10 years to support Indigenous priorities and complementary federal support, for a total of $198.6 billion over 10 years. These investments will further help provide Canadians with health care that includes access to high-quality family health services when they need them, including in rural and remote areas and for underserved communities; a resilient and supported health workforce that provides them high-quality, effective, and safe health services when they need them; and access to timely, equitable, and quality mental health, substance use, and addictions services to support their well-being.[46]

United Kingdom

In March of 2020, the UK government announced a £5 million grant, administered by Mind (a charity in England), to fund additional services for people struggling with their mental well-being during the pandemic. In May 2020, the government announced a further £4.2 million for mental health charities, such as Samaritans, Young Minds, and Bipolar UK, to continue to support people experiencing mental health challenges throughout the outbreak.[47]

In 2022, the government issued a call for evidence to inform a new, 10-year cross-government mental health and well-being plan. In January of 2023 the government announced it will publish a major conditions strategy that will include mental health. The government has said a joined-up strategy will ensure that mental health conditions are considered alongside physical health conditions, addressing the ongoing mental healthcare crisis involving communities and governments.[48]

The government's "Build Back Better: Our Plan for Health and Social Care" (September 2021) policy paper aims to address the challenges caused by the pandemic on the health and social care systems. It recognizes "the pandemic affected mental health, with unprecedented demands placed on staff and the public as a whole." In addition to funding commitments, wider changes to support the social care system are proposed, including investments to fund mental health and well-being resources.[49]

Spain

A 2021–2024 Mental Health and COVID-19 Action Plan was implemented, which had €100 million allocated from the Government of Spain, and was formulated "in response to the emergency caused by the impact of the COVID pandemic on mental health and in response to the Opinion of the Reconstruction Commission." The improvement of mental health care at all levels of the National Health System—both in hospital and primary care—is one of the main measures included in the new plan, together with the promotion of specialized health care training in mental health, awareness raising and the fight against stigmatization, the prevention of addictive behaviors, the promotion of emotional well-being—focusing on children, adolescents, and other vulnerable groups such as women and the elderly—and the improvement of prevention, detection, and care of suicidal tendencies.[50]

Italy

In March of 2020, the Italian government launched a national mental health service intended to combat the rise of mental distress in Italy by funding multiple government programs and free mental health services (servizi di salute metale). The program works with institutions and regional associations to provide free emergency help from psychanalysts and psychologists. Italy has also announced plans to introduce a €10 million psychologist bonus to help people access mental health services as part of the new milleproroghe amendment bill.

Addressing the ongoing mental healthcare crisis involves communities, governments, healthcare professionals, and mental health providers collaborating and devising interventions that are obtainable, efficient, and effective. It is a multifaceted problem that requires multiple solutions to best serve clients and maintain mental wellness in our countries. Developing adequate community-based mental health care programs is not a single, clear-cut process that will work efficiently in every country. Behavioral and mental health systems that function efficiently in the United States may not meet mental health care recipients'

BOX 8.2 A Critical Thinking Synopsis—Do You Agree?

It is a well-documented, evidence-based fact that trauma impacts mental well-being. For prevention strategies to be effective, a cultural ideology shift needs to occur worldwide that encompasses a belief of intolerance of all forms of abuse (bullying, gender discrimination, domestic abuse, intimate partner violence, coercive control) and holds harm doers accountable.

Regarding individuals who experience SMI, the exploitation, bullying, and discrimination need to be eradicated worldwide.

And the additional social stressors that deter recovery need to stop to sustain mental well-being within communities.

needs in Mexico or Taiwan. The solutions to addressing mental wellness are as diverse as each country's infrastructure and need to be evaluated with the problem-solving processes.

Main Points

1. Today, modern hospital settings include BHUs that are used for short-term stays inside general hospitals; these units are used for the stabilization of acute psychiatric episodes.
2. Initial licenses for a psychiatric-based treatment entity are issued when the state licensing division receives a completed application with appropriate monetary fees, and the institution meets all the state-mandated requirements for the operation of a psychiatric/behavioral unit or psychiatric hospital.
3. There are several studies that have been conducted that demonstrate that a psychiatric unit's physical environment can be directly correlated to the levels and episodes of aggression demonstrated by clients.
4. Inpatient psychiatric services should be part of an overall plan of care, supporting a coordinated effort between the patient, family, treatment team, and outpatient service providers.
5. The overwhelming evidence that there is a definitive connection between mental and physical health supports the integration of mental health services into the primary care setting.
6. Trauma-informed care is the delivery of services that promote recovery and healing from trauma rather than practices that retraumatize individuals.
7. Technology utilization in mental health treatment (e-mental health) ranges from support services, data collection, monitoring progress, tracking behaviors, and understanding mental well-being. Benefits related to e-mental health include being easily accessible, filling service gaps, saving the practitioner's time, providing flexibility, and being cost-effective.
8. Governments across the globe have recognized that the COVID-19 pandemic exposed and exacerbated the already broken mental healthcare delivery systems that exist in the majority of countries.

Notes

1. Legal Action Center, The Medicaid IMD exclusion: An overview and opportunities for reform, http://lac.org/assets/files/IMD_exclusion_fact_sheet.pdf (accessed April 20, 2020).
2. Loveridge, Melissa (2021), *Locals rally to urge Bozeman Health to add inpatient psychiatric health care*, https://www.bozemandailychronicle.com/news/health/

locals-rally-to-urge-bozeman-health-to-add-inpatient-psychiatric-health-care/article_b7f2f264-7b12-57ed-ac44-fb15af401491.html (accessed August 26, 2023).

3. Loveridge, Melissa (2021), *Locals rally to urge Bozeman Health to add inpatient psychiatric health care,* https://www.bozemandailychronicle.com/news/health/locals-rally-to-urge-bozeman-health-to-add-inpatient-psychiatric-health-care/article_b7f2f264-7b12-57ed-ac44-fb15af401491.html (accessed August 26, 2023).
4. Legal Information Institute, Wyoming current rules and regulations for licensure of psychiatric hospitals, https://www.law.cornell.edu/regulations/wyoming/agency (accessed April 20, 2020).
5. Legal Information Institute, Wyoming current rules and regulations for licensure of psychiatric hospitals, https://www.law.cornell.edu/regulations/wyoming/agency (accessed April 20, 2020).
6. van der Schaaf, P.S. et al. (2013), Impact of the physical environment of psychiatric wards on the use of seclusion, *The British Journal of Psychiatry,* https://www.cambridge.org/core/journals/the-british-journal-of-psychiatry/article/impact-of-the-physical-environment-of-psychiatric-wards-on-the-use-of-seclusion/ECF01A965156AF94A632E8436F13FD9D (accessed March 3, 2020), pp. 1–6.
7. van der Schaaf, P.S. et al. (2013), Impact of the physical environment of psychiatric wards on the use of seclusion, *The British Journal of Psychiatry,* https://www.cambridge.org/core/journals/the-british-journal-of-psychiatry/article/impact-of-the-physical-environment-of-psychiatric-wards-on-the-use-of-seclusion/ECF01A965156AF94A632E8436F13FD9D (accessed March 3, 2020), pp. 1–6.
8. Bolton, Aaron (2023), *Her husband died after stay at Montana State Hospital. She wants answers,* Montana Public Radio, NPR News, https://www.npr.org/sections/health-shots/2023/03/02/1160480706/her-husband-died-after-stay-at-montana-state-hospital-she-wants-answers#:~:text=Jennifer%20Mitchell%2C%20the%20woman%20whose%20husband%20died%20shortly,worries%20more%20patients%20will%20die%20at%20the%20facility (accessed August 27, 2023).
9. Legal Information Institute, Wyoming current rules and regulations for licensure of psychiatric hospitals, https://www.law.cornell.edu/regulations/wyoming/agency (accessed April 20, 2020).
10. Medicare Benefit Policy Manual (2018), Inpatient psychiatric facility services Centers for Medicare and Medicaid Services, Chapter Two, https://www.cms.gov/Regulations-and-Guidance/Guidance/Manuals/Downloads/bp102c02.pdf (accessed April 20, 2020), pp. 1–18.
11. Open Minds (2022), *2022 turn over at behavioral health facilities averages more than 30%,* https://openminds.com/market-intelligence/news/2022-turnover-at-behavioral-health-facilities-averages-more-than-30/ (accessed August 25, 2023).
12. Texas Center for Nursing Workforce Studies (2019), *Hospital nurse staffing study: State mental health facilities,* https://www.dshs.texas.gov/cns/cnws/hnss/2019/2019-hnss-state-mental-health-facilities.pdf. (accessed May 13, 2022), pp. 1–3.
13. Center for Medicare and Medicaid Services (2018), Inpatient psychiatric facility services Centers for Medicare and Medicaid Services, Medicare Benefit Policy Manual, Chapter Two, pp. 1–18.
14. WHO (2019), *Facilities data by country,* Global Health Observatory, https://apps.who.int/gho/data/view.main.MHFACv (accessed August 26, 2023).
15. Our World in Data (2017), *Mental health units in general hospitals,* httpd://ourworldindata.org/grapher/mental-health-units-in-general-hospitals (accessed August 26, 2023).

16. Cronin, T. (2017), *A comparison of mental health legislation in five developed countries: A narrative review*, Cambridge University Press, https://www.cambridge.org/core/journals/irish-journal-of-psychological-medicine/article/comparison-of-mental-health-legislation-in-five-developed-countries-a-narrative-review/1043291DBE9B8D24480D738D47E1BAD6 (accessed August 26, 2023).
17. Mental Health Services for Children and Adolescents, *Family guide: Children's mental health services*, Texas Department of State Health Services, http://www.dshs.state.tx.us/mhsa/mh-child-adolescent-services (accessed May 5, 2020), pp. 1–16.
18. Mental Health Services for Children and Adolescents, *Family guide: Children's mental health services*, Texas Department of State Health Services, http://www.dshs.state.tx.us/mhsa/mh-child-adolescent-services (accessed May 5, 2020), pp. 1–16.
19. Kowakchuk, Alicia, DO et al. (2022), Anxiety disorders in children and adolescents, *Am Fam Physician* 106(6), https://www.aafp.org/pubs/afp/issues/2022/1200/anxiety-disorders-children-adolescents.html, pp. 657–664.
20. WHO (2021), *Mental health of adolescents*, https://www.who.int/news-room/fact-sheets/detail/adolescent-mental-health (accessed August 25, 2023).
21. Unutzer, Jurgen, MD et al. (2013), *The collaborative care model: An approach for integrating physical and mental health care in Medicaid health homes*, Center for Health Care Strategies, https://www.chcs.org/resource/the-collaborative-care-model-an-approach-for-integrating-physical-and-mental-health-care-in-medicaid-health-homes (accessed November 12, 2021).
22. Unutzer, Jurgen, MD et al. (2013), *The collaborative care model: An approach for integrating physical and mental health care in Medicaid health homes*, https://www.chcs.org/resource/the-collaborative-care-model-an-approach-for-integrating-physical-and-mental-health-care-in-medicaid-health-homes (accessed November 12, 2021).
23. National Council on Behavioral Health (2020), *How to manage trauma*, https://www.thenationalcouncil.org/resources/how-to-manage-trauma/ (accessed November 12, 2021).
24. Robeznieks, Andis (2121), *Why doctors must grasp patient's context in trauma-informed care*, https://www.ama-assn.org/delivering-care/health-equity/why-doctors-must-grasp-patients-contex-in-trauma-informed-care
25. California Academy of Family Physicians (2010), CAFP launches family medicine initiative on trauma-informed care, https://www.familydocs.org/aces (accessed November 12, 2021).
26. Sweeney, Colm et al. (2021), Can chatbots help support a person's mental health? Perceptions and views from mental healthcare professionals and experts, *ACM Trans. Comp. Healthcare*, 2(3), Article 25, https://doi.org/10.1145/3453175 (accessed May 9, 2022).[27] Mental Health Foundation (2022), *eMEN digital mental health European project*, https://cpmr.mentalhealth.org.uk/sp/node/2092. (accessed May 9, 2022).
27. American Psychiatric Association (2018), *APA and ATA release new telemental health guide*, https://www.psychiatry.org/psychiatrists/practice/telepsychiatry/blog/apa-and-ata-release-new-telemental-health-guide (accessed August 25, 2023).
28. Abraham, Amit et al. (2021), Telemental health use in the COVID-19 pandemic: A scoping review and evidence gap mapping, *Front Psychiatry*, 12, 748069, https://www.ncbi.nlm.nih.gov/pmc/articles/PMC8606591/ (accessed August 26, 2023).
29. The White House (2022), *Fact sheet: President Biden to announce strategy to address our national mental health crisis, as part of unity agenda in his first State of the Union*, https://www.whitehouse.gov/briefing/-room/statements-releases/2022/03/01/

fact-sheet-president-biden-to-announce-strategy-to-address-our-national-mental-health-crisis-as-part-of-unity-agenda-in-his-first-state-of-the-union/ (accessed August 25, 2023).

30. The White House (2022), *Fact sheet: President Biden to announce strategy to address our national mental health crisis, as part of unity agenda in his first State of the Union*, https:/www.whitehouse.gov/briefing /-room/statements-releases/2022/03/01/fact-sheet-president-biden-to-announce-strategy-to-address-our-national-mental-health-crisis-as-part-of-unity-agenda-in-his-first-state-of-the-union/ (accessed August 25, 2023).
31. The White House (2022), *Fact sheet: President Biden to announce strategy to address our national mental health crisis, as part of unity agenda in his first State of the Union*, https:/www.whitehouse.gov/briefing /-room/statements-releases/2022/03/01/fact-sheet-president-biden-to-announce-strategy-to-address-our-national-mental-health-crisis-as-part-of-unity-agenda-in-his-first-state-of-the-union/ (accessed August 25, 2023).
32. National Governors Association (2023), *Governors top health priorities in 2023 State of the State addresses*, https://www.nga.org/news/commentary/governors-top-health-prioritiesin-2023-state-of-the-state-addresses/ (accessed August 27, 2023).
33. The White House (2022), *Fact sheet: President Biden to announce strategy to address our national mental health crisis, as part of unity agenda in his first State of the Union*, https:/www.whitehouse.gov/briefing /-room/statements-releases/2022/03/01/fact-sheet-president-biden-to-announce-strategy-to-address-our-national-mental-health-crisis-as-part-of-unity-agenda-in-his-first-state-of-the-union/ (accessed August 25, 2023).
34. National Governors Association (2023), *Governors top health priorities in 2023 State of the State addresses*, https://www.nga.org/news/commentary/governors-top-health-prioritiesin-2023-state-of-the-state-addresses/ (accessed August 27, 2023).
35. The White House (2022), *Fact sheet: President Biden to announce strategy to address our national mental health crisis, as part of unity agenda in his first State of the Union*, https:/www.whitehouse.gov/briefing /-room/statements-releases/2022/03/01/fact-sheet-president-biden-to-announce-strategy-to-address-our-national-mental-health-crisis-as-part-of-unity-agenda-in-his-first-state-of-the-union/ (accessed August 25, 2023).
36. The White House (2023), *Fact sheet: Biden-Harris administration announces new actions to tackle nation's mental health crisis*, https://www.whitehouse.gov/briefing-room/statements-releases/2023/05/18/fact-sheet-biden-harris-administration-announces-new-actions-to-tackle-nations-mental-health-crisis/ (accessed August 25, 2023).
37. The White House (2023), *Fact sheet: Biden-Harris administration announces new actions to tackle nation's mental health crisis*, https://www.whitehouse.gov/briefing-room/statements-releases/2023/05/18/fact-sheet-biden-harris-administration-announces-new-actions-to-tackle-nations-mental-health-crisis/ (accessed August 25, 2023).
38. National Governors Association (2023), *Governors top health priorities in 2023 State of the State addresses*, https://www.nga.org/news/commentary/governors-top-health-prioritiesin-2023-state-of-the-state-addresses/ (accessed August 27, 2023)
39. The White House (2023), *Fact sheet: Biden-Harris administration announces new actions to tackle nation's mental health crisis*, https://www.whitehouse.gov/briefing-room/statements-releases/2023/05/18/fact-sheet-biden-harris-administration-announces-new-actions-to-tackle-nations-mental-health-crisis/ (accessed August 25, 2023).
40. The White House (2023), *Fact sheet: Biden-Harris administration announces new actions to tackle nation's mental health crisis*, https://www.whitehouse.gov/briefing-room/statements-releases/2023/05/18/fact-sheet-biden-harris-administration-announces-new-actions-to-tackle-nations-mental-health-crisis/ (accessed August 25, 2023).

41. The White House (2023), *Fact sheet: Biden-Harris administration announces new actions to tackle nation's mental health crisis,* https://www.whitehouse.gov/briefing-room/statements-releases/2023/05/18/fact-sheet-biden-harris-administration-announces-new-actions-to-tackle-nations-mental-health-crisis/ (accessed August 25, 2023).
42. The White House (2023), *Fact sheet: Biden-Harris administration announces new actions to tackle nation's mental health crisis,* https://www.whitehouse.gov/briefing-room/statements-releases/2023/05/18/fact-sheet-biden-harris-administration-announces-new-actions-to-tackle-nations-mental-health-crisis/ (accessed August 25, 2023).
43. National Governors Association (2023), *Governors top health priorities in 2023 State of the State addresses,* https://www.nga.org/news/commentary/governors-top-health-prioritiesin-2023-state-of-the-state-addresses/ (accessed August 27, 2023).
44. National Governors Association (2023), *Governors top health priorities in 2023 State of the State addresses,* https://www.nga.org/news/commentary/governors-top-health-prioritiesin-2023-state-of-the-state-addresses/ (accessed August 27, 2023).
45. Government of Canada (2023), *Working together to improve healthcare for Canadians,* https://www.canada.ca/en/health-canada/news/2023/02/working-togeth-er-to-improve-health-care-for-canadians.html (accessed August 25, 2023).
46. Garrett, Katherine (2023), *Mental health policy in England,* House of Commons, https://researchbriefings. files.parliament.uk/documents/CBP-7547/CBP-7547.pdf (accessed August 25, 2023).
47. Garrett, Katherine (2023), *Mental health policy in England,* House of Commons, https://researchbriefings. files.parliament.uk/documents/CBP-7547/CBP-7547.pdf (accessed August 25, 2023).
48. Garrett, Katherine (2023), *Mental health policy in England,* House of Commons, https://researchbriefings. files.parliament.uk/documents/CBP-7547/CBP-7547.pdf (accessed August 25, 2023).
49. Moncloa Palace, Madrid (2021), *The government unveils the 2021–2024 mental health and COVID-19 action plan to address the impact of the pandemic,* https://www.lamoncloa.gob.es/lang/en/presidente/news/paginas/2021/20211009_mental-health- plan.aspx#:~:-text=The%20improvement%20of%20Mental%20Health%20Care%20at%20all,of%20prevention%2C%20detection%20and%20care%20of%20suicidal%20tendencies (accessed August 25, 2023).
50. Allaby, Elaine (2022), *How Italy is addressing its pandemic induced mental health crisis,* https://www.thelocal.it/20220218/how-is-italy-addressing-its-pandemic-induced-mental-health-crisis (accessed August 26, 2023).

Credits

Fig. 8.1: Data Source: https://www.dshs.texas.gov/sites/default/files/chs/cnws/HNS-S/2019/2019-HNSS-State-Mental-Health-Facilities.pdf.

APPENDIX

Supplemental Psychiatric Material

As more knowledge was obtained with regard to the human brain and its functionality, there became an increase in awareness of the lack of necessity to institutionalize all individuals who experience mental conditions.

In the history of psychiatry, the earliest foundation of psychology can be traced back to the ancient Greeks, yet this field of medicine was not fully developed as a separate discipline until the 1800s. The term "psychiatry" came into existence in 1808 when Johann Christian Reil (a German physician) developed and expanded on the mental health field.[1] Psychiatry is a term that depicts a branch of medicine that is dedicated to the treatment and study of psychological conditions. And psychology is defined as the scientific and academic study of the mind, encompassing an individual's behaviors and the thoughts, feelings, and motivations connected to those behaviors.

The concept of the mind and body being separate entities that coexist in functionality was introduced as "dualism" in the 17th century by French philosopher Rene Descartes.[2] Physiological studies of the human brain, over the years, have also contributed to the scientific methodologies used to study human thought and behavior in modern psychology. Today, we know that mental health can affect physical health and vice versa, so I believe the concept of holism is applicable when it comes to mental health treatment services.

Psychiatry has evolved and progressed in many countries; in India, the field of psychology as a separate entity was established in 1916 at Calcutta University through the Department of Experimental Psychology. The first psychological laboratory was established in Japan by Yujiro Motora at the University of Tokyo in 1903. During the Golden Age of Islam, Muhammad ibn Zakariya al-Razi (physician, philosopher, and scientist) was among the first globally to write about mental illness and psychotherapy. Vittorio Benussi, a professor of psychology at the University of Padova, Italy, established a lab to study vision and time perception in 1919. And Dalhousie University (1838) offered the first psychology course in Canada; Thomas McCulloch taught the class.

The field of psychiatry can be subdivided into three categories: mental illness, learning disorders, and personality disorders. Learning disorders encompass unknown factors that affect the brain's ability to receive and process information. Mental illnesses are any illness of a psychological origin that exhibits emotional and/or behavioral symptomatology. And personality disorders typically are personality types that deviate from social expectations in relation to other human beings.

Psychological Theories

There have been many psychological theories formulated and used throughout the years to assist in understanding human thought, development, and behavior. Over the years, some of these theories have remained widely accepted within the profession, and others have been discarded because of proof of inaccuracy. We will explore a few of the established theories to provide a framework of understanding encompassing the thought processes of psychological field development.

The first two theories related to psychology were structuralism and functionalism. Structuralism focuses on analyzing elements of mental experiences (sensations, mental images, feelings) and how they form more complex experiences. Functionalism was introduced by William James, an American psychologist, through his book *The Principles of Psychology*, released in 1950. The basis of thought related to functionalism was that behaviors worked to help individuals live in their environment. Behaviorism is a theory based on the concept that all behaviors are acquired through conditioning. Behavioral techniques are still widely practiced in therapeutic settings in modern psychiatry, including operant and classical conditioning. Cognitive theories are focused on internal states, such as motivation, problem-solving, decision-making, thinking, and attention. Specific areas addressed under this theory are memory, attention, right- and left-brain dominance, perceptual organization, cognitive development, and intelligence. Developmental theories focus on human growth, development, and learning; these theories provide a framework for insight into individuals and societal behaviors and thoughts.

Humanists' theories focus on the basic goodness of human beings, addressing Maslow's hierarchy of needs. Personality theories are grounded in the patterns of thoughts, feelings, and behaviors that make individuals unique. Separate entities that are examined in personalities are defense mechanisms, archetypes, psychogenic needs, neurotic needs, and personality traits. Social psychology theories assist in understanding social behavior that can encompass actor-observer bias, altruism, bystander effect, compliance, conformity, heroism, leadership, love, and reciprocity. Learning theories explain how individuals learn and acquire new knowledge. And psychological theories provide a broad base of understanding about the hows and whys of human behavior and generate a basis for future research. There are many different approaches (perspectives) in contemporary psychiatry, and each perspective can hold several beliefs. This process of examining the many different aspects of psychology unfolds something different in each entity to assist in our understanding of human behavior.

Psychiatrists and Psychologists

Carl Gustav Jung, born in 1875, was a Swiss psychiatrist who graduated from the University of Zurich in 1903. His major contribution to the field of psychology is that he founded the school of analytical psychology, which aims to analyze human psychology in its wholeness through the integration of unconscious forces and motivations present in the human subconscious mind. The theories he contributed to the field of psychology include the following:

- The concept of introversion and extroversion
- The archetypes and synchronicity[2]

In 1906, Jung published *Studies in Word Association* and sent a copy to psychiatrist Sigmund Freud, which initiated a friendship that lasted approximately 6 years. The two men influenced each other intellectually and attended many seminars together. When Dr. Jung began his work on the *Psychology of the Unconscious,* strain developed in the Freud/Jung relationship because of opposing views on libido and religion.

Sigmund Freud

Born in 1856, Sigmund Schlomo Freud is considered the father of psychoanalysis. Dr. Freud was an Austrian psychiatrist who graduated from the University of Vienna. His intellect encompassed an ability to learn eight different languages fluently, including Latin, Hebrew, Greek, German, English, French, Spanish, and Italian. The collection of theoretical contributions developed by Dr. Freud, relating to the mind and the mysteries locked within, transformed the field of psychology and how individuals viewed the brain and its functional processes. His major published works include the following:

- *The Interpretation of Dreams*
- *The Psychopathology of Everyday Life*
- *The Ego and the Id*[3]

Dr. Freud spent every Wednesday lecturing on his newly formulated theories, which led to the development of the Wednesday Psychological Society that grew over time and by 1908 was developed into a formal group called The International Psychoanalytical Congress. As his popularity grew, Dr. Freud was subsequently named president of the American Psychoanalytical Society when the group was formulated in 1911.

When Adolf Hitler was appointed as chancellor of Germany in 1933, many of Dr. Freud's publications were burned and destroyed. As a result, Sigmund Freud had to flee Vienna for Britain with his family to avoid Nazi brutality. Dr. Freud's work began to decline in popularity in the 1950s because of his blatant contrast of perceptions about gender equality. He marginalized his perceptions of female sexuality by extending his views of male sexuality to women, viewing women as simply castrated males.

Freud's theory of penis envy, which is the jealousy little girls feel toward boys and the resentment toward their mothers for not having a penis; according to Freud led to underdeveloped superegos, implying that women will always be morally inferior to men. Early sexologists agreed with Freud that women were passive in sex and simply engaged in the activity to produce children. His willful ignorance of the acceptance of female sexuality and how it may differ from male sexuality continues to influence some sexologists and psychologists in modern times.

Dr. Freud was an early user of cocaine, and it is believed that it abated his mental and physical problems. He suffered from frequent bouts of depression and self-medicated with coca leaves to manage his anxiety. There continues to be some debate with regard to his substance utilization and whether it influenced his perceptions and the formulation of his psychological theories. Many argue that he wrote his article "Uber Coca" in 1884 and stopped his cocaine addiction in 1896 with the publication of *The Aetiology of Hysteria*, where the term "psychoanalysis" was first introduced and described.[4] He fought a battle with jaw cancer that entailed 33 surgeries and ended his life with an administered morphine-induced death in 1939.

Herman Rorschach

Dr. Rorschach was a Swiss psychiatrist who developed the projective test called the Rorschach inkblot test. The test is a set of 10 inkblot cards that are supposed to reveal an individual's subconscious personality traits. Dr. Rorschach completed a study using the abstract inkblot cards and published his findings in 1921 through the monograph *Psychodiagnostik*. He was deeply fascinated by klecksography, the art of making fanciful inkblot images.

Today, these tests are used in various branches, such as military training and career counseling. There has been controversy over the utilization of these tests. The Board of Trustees of the Society for Personality Assessment released a position paper in support of the inkblot testing based on data collected in 2001.[5] Dr. Rorschach earned his doctor of medicine degree from the University of Zurich in 1912. He did not live to see the success of his development; he died at the age of 37 in 1922 from peritonitis.

Ronald David Laing

Dr. Laing was a Scottish psychiatrist who worked extensively on a number of mental illnesses in the 1950s and 1960s, including psychosis and schizophrenia. What set him apart from other psychiatrists in his field is he based his diagnosis and treatment on the feelings expressed by his patients. Dr. Laing believed that the treatment of mentally ill clients must be based on interpersonal therapy, including clients speaking freely to the therapist. He contributed several published works to the field of psychiatry, including the following:

- *The Divided Self*
- *Sanity, Madness, and the Family*

- *The Politics of Experience and the Bird of Paradise*
- *Wisdom, Madness, and Folly*[6]

In 1988, Dr. Laing had to discontinue his practice because of alcoholism and clinical depression.

Alfred Adler

Dr. Adler graduated from the University of Vienna in 1895 with a medical degree and began his practice as an ophthalmologist, later switching to general medical practice. By 1902, he had an increased interest in the field of psychiatry. He spent some of his psychiatric career with Dr. Sigmund Freud but had a disagreement with some of Freud's theories and terminated the relationship after a short period. In 1912, Dr. Adler founded the Society of Individual Psychology based on his concept of the inferiority complex.[7] He believed that human beings strived for superiority over others and that this drive was the motivating force behind human behaviors, emotions, and thoughts, often referred to as Adlerian psychology.

Dr. Adler relocated to the United States in the 1930s to fill a professor position at Long Island College of Medicine. He also toured frequently, lecturing on his psychological theories. During one of these tours in 1937, he suffered a fatal heart attack. Seventy-four years after his death (2011), his cremated remains were found in a crematorium in Edinburgh, Scotland, and returned to Vienna, Austria.[8]

Wilhelm Wundt

Known as the father of experimental psychology, Dr. Wundt founded the Institute for Experimental Psychology in 1879 at the University of Leipzig in Germany.[9] This was the first laboratory explicitly for psychological studies, with the emphasis and focus being placed on data collection using measurement and control. The philosophies that evolved from the laboratory involved three specific systems: voluntarism, structuralism, and introspection. Voluntarism is described as the process of organizing the mind. Structuralism is the analysis of the basic elements that constitute the mind. And introspection is a highly practiced form of self-examination. His work was a study of perceptual processes, including thoughts, images and feelings and stimulated interest in current cognitive psychology practices.

Experiments and Research

Over the years, there have been numerous classic studies and experiments in the field of psychology. Some of the experiments have been deemed controversial within society and the medical community. We will examine a few of the most identified fascinating experiments and their results.

Social Isolation

The social isolation experiments, conducted by Harry Harlow in 1958, examined young rhesus monkeys exposed to a wire and a cloth simulation of a mother monkey, with the wire monkey in one group providing nourishment to the babies. The results of the experiment demonstrated that the infant monkeys spent the majority of their time with the cloth simulator of a mother monkey, and in the one experimental group, the monkeys used the wire-developed mother monkey "only" for nourishment. This experiment demonstrated that "nature and nurture" are both required for healthy development and that contact comfort is necessary for the development of affectional response.[10]

Little Albert

By today's standards, the "Little Albert" experiment performed in 1920 by behaviorist John B. Watson is deemed unethical. The experiment was performed to determine if fear was innate or a conditioned response. A 9-month-old child was exposed to a white rat with a loud noise simultaneously conducted during the visual exposure of the animal. The experiment elicited the emotion of fear and crying from the child. Over a period of time, the child began to exhibit fear and crying, while being exposed to just the white rat, and no loud noise simultaneously performed. The conditioned response elicited from the child in the experiment was fear. Little Albert also started to generalize his fear response to anything fluffy or white (or both). It is believed that Albert Barger was the baby used in the experiment: he lived a long, happy life, but he did have an aversion to animals. Albert Barger passed away in 2007.[11]

Stanford Prison

The Stanford Prison Experiment, conducted by psychology professor Philip Zimbardo in 1971, focused on the psychological effects of becoming a prisoner or a prison guard in a correctional facility setting. In the experiment, 24 males were used in a mock prison situated in the basement of the Stanford psychology building for a period of 7 to 14 days.

Participants in the study adapted to their roles well beyond expectations; prison guards subjected the prisoners to psychological torture, and many of the prisoners passively accepted the psychological abuse. Philip Zimbardo, acting as the superintendent of the prison, did not attempt to stop the psychological tactics portrayed in the simulated prison. Because approximately one third of the guards became sadistically cruel during the experiment, the process was abruptly terminated after 6 days.

It is argued that the results of the experiment demonstrate that situational occurrences of behaviors can be developed because of conformity psychology versus individualized personality characteristics. The experiment has been used to illustrate the cognitive dissonance theory and the power of authority in abuse situations. The lesson of the Stanford Experiment isn't that any random human being is capable of descending into sadism and tyranny. It's that certain institutions and environments demand those behaviors and that people are shaped by preexisting norms and patterns of behavior.[12]

Learned Helplessness

The 1965 learned helplessness experiment conducted by psychologists Mark Seligman and Steve Maier used three groups of dogs in the experimental process. All of the animals were placed in harnesses, and two of the groups were subjected to electrical shocks while being harnessed together.

Group 1 dogs were not subjected to electrical shocks and demonstrated no harm from the experiment. Group 2 dogs were given electrical shocks that could be terminated by pushing a lever, and Group 3 dogs were given random electrical shocks that could not be terminated. The animals in Group 3 demonstrated signs of clinical depression and "learned helplessness" because, over a period of time, the dogs did not even attempt to find a way to terminate the abuse. Steve Maier, 30 years later, conducted a series of experiments that led to the conclusion that it was the release of serotonin from the dorsal raphe nucleus that was responsible for the behavioral effects.[13]

David Reimer

A case involving a young boy named David Reimer, who had his penis burned off during a circumcision procedure at 8 months old, elicited controversy regarding the psychologist John Money. David Reimer's parents consulted a psychologist after the accident to obtain assistance on how to help their son.

Psychologist John Money convinced the parents to obtain a sex change operation for their son so he could prove that nurture, not nature, determined gender identity. David became Brenda, but the results of the sex change operation had consequences that were confusing for the child because the child possessed a male brain.

At age 14, David's parents told him the truth about the events that occurred when he was a baby, and David decided to become a male again. Because of the confusing aspects of David Reimer's life surrounding gender identity, he committed suicide at the age of 38. The case of David Reimer seems to refute the nurture theory—that is, the idea that gender identity is due solely to social effects.[14]

Psychiatry is still evolving today; one example is the utilization of neuroscience and brain imaging studies in an attempt to better understand violent behavior. The Stanford Prison and the learned helplessness experiments offered some insight into specific behaviors during their time frame of conduction, but technology has advanced in so many spectrums, allowing for an even deeper understanding of human behavior that can eventually assist in devising effective treatment modalities.

Notes

1. Society for Recognition of Famous People (2020), *The famous people: Psychiatrists*, http://thefamouspeople.com/psychiatrists.php (accessed July 6, 2020).
2. Boeree, George Dr. (2006), *Carl Jung (1875–1961) personality theories*, Psychology Department Shippensburg University, https://webspace.ship.edu/cgboer/perscontents.html (accessed March 16, 2020).
3. Bradford, Alina (2016), *Sigmund Freud: Life, work, & theories*, Live Science, http://www.livescience.com, (accessed March 16, 2020).
4. Nuland, Sherwin (2011), Sigmund Freud's cocaine years, *New York Times*, https://www.nytimes.com/2011/07/24/book/review/an-anatomy-of-addiction-by-howard-markel/html (accessed December 18, 2019).
5. Society of Personality Assessment (2005), The status of the Rorschach in clinical and forensic practice: An official statement by the Board of Trustees of the Society for Personality Testing, *Journal of Personality Assessment*, 85(2), https://www.tandfonline.com/doi/full/10.1080/00223891.2017.1394869#:~:text=The%20Rorschach%20Institute%20began%20as%20an,Wolfson%29%2C%20and%20a%20treasurer%20%28Gladys%20Tallman%29.&text=The%20Rorschach%20Institute%20began,a%20treasurer%20%28Gladys%20Tallman%29.&text=Institute%20began%20as%20an,Wolfson%29%2C%20and%20a%20treasurer (accessed December 18, 2019), pp. 219–237.
6. Laing Society (2002), *R.D. Laing—biography*, http://www.laingsociety.org (accessed December 18, 2019).
7. International Association of Individual Psychology (2012), *Alfred Adler*, https://www.adler.iaip.net (accessed November 26, 2019).
8. Adler University, Alfred Adler (1870–1937), http://adler.edu/alfred-adler-history (accessed November 20, 2019).
9. Leipzig University, History of Psychology in Leipzig, Germany, Department of Psychology, http://www.psychologie.biphaps.uni-leipzig.de (accessed October 18, 2019).
10. Fung, Janice (2013), Harlow's experiments on attachment in monkeys: Theories of psychological development, https://www.slideshare.net/janfu1/psychology-harlows-experiments-on-attachment-in-monkeys (accessed May 10, 2019).
11. Thomson, Helen (2014), Baby used in notorious fear experiment is lost no more, *New Scientist Magazine*, https://newscientist.com/article/dn26307-baby-used-in-notorious-fear-experiment-is-lost-no-more (accessed August 18, 2019).
12. Konnikova, Maria (2015), The real lessons of the Stanford prison experiment, *The New Yorker*, https://www.newyorker.com/science/maria-konnikova/the-real-lessons-of-the-stanford-prison (accessed September 15, 2019).
13. Dingfelder, Sadie (2009), Old problem, new tools: One of the psychologists who discovered learned helplessness returns, *Monitor on Psychology*, *40*(9). https://www.apa.org/monitor/2009/10/helplessness
14. Schillo, Keit (2011), *Nature or nurture: The case of the boy who became a girl*. National Center for Case Study Teaching in Science, https://sciencecases.lib.buffalo.edu/files/gender-reassignent.pdf (accessed November 18, 2019).

BIBLIOGRAPHY

Abramson, A. (2022). Children's mental health is in crisis. *Monitor on Psychology, 53*(1). https://www.apa.org/monitor/2022/01/special-childrens-mental-health

Adams County Historical Society. (n.d.). *Hastings State Hospital.* http://www.rootsweb.ancestry.com/-asylums/hastings_nb/index.html

Adler University. (n.d.). *Alfred Adler (1870–1937).* http://adler.edu/alfred-adler-history

Alhaj, H., & MCC Psych. (2019). *A practical guide to the use of seclusion in mental health settings.* National Association of Psychiatric Intensive Care. https://napicu.org.uk/wo-content/uploads/2019/04/HAMID-BAP-NAPICU-Cambridge

Alliance for Consumer Education. (2020). *How prevalent is inhalant abuse in the United States?* https://www.consumered.org/programs/inhalant-abuse-prevention/data-research#

American Academy of Pediatrics. (2021). *AAP-AACAP-CHA; declaration of a national emergency in child and adolescent mental health.* https://www.aap.org/en/advocacy/child-and-adolescent-healthy-mental-development/aap-aacap-cha-declaration-of-a-national-emergency

American Experience. (n.d.). *Primary sources: Insulin coma therapy.* https://www.pbs.com/f/insulin+com+therapy.doc

Appleton, V. E. (1967). Psychiatry in Canada a century ago. *Canadian Psychiatric Association Journal, 12*(4). 345–361. https://www.journals.sagepub.com/doi/abs/10.117/070674376701200402

Aschbrenner, K., Grabowski, D. C., Cai, S., Bartels, S. J., & Mor, V. (2011). Nursing homes admissions and long-stay conversions among persons with and without serious mental illness. *Journal of Aging and Social Policy,* 23(3), 286–304. https://pubmed.ncbi.nlm.nih.gov/21740203/

Association for Community Mental Health Centers. (2021). *Why is funding for community mental health centers (CMHCs) important.* https://www.acmhck.org/resources/why-is-funding-for-comunity-mental-health-centers-important

Asylum Projects. (2021). *Charenton.* https://www.asylumprojects.org/index.php.title-charenton

Ayusi-Mateos, J. L. (2021). Informing the response to COVID-19 in Spain: Priorities for mental health research. *Rev Psiquiatr Salud Ment, 14*(2), 79–82. https://doi.org/10.1016/j.rpsmen.2021.04.001

Barbui, C., Papola, D., & Saraceneo, B. (2018). Forty years without mental hospitals in Italy. *International Journal of Mental Health Systems,* 12(43). https://doi.org/10.1186/s13033-018-0223-1

Beck, A., Page, C., Buche, J., Rittman, D., & Gaiser, M. (2018). *Estimating the distribution of the U.S. psychiatric subspecialist workforce.* School of Public Health Behavioral Science Workforce Research Center, University of Michigan, https://www.behavioralhealthworkforce.org/project/distribution-of-psychiatric-subspecialties-in-the-behavioral-health-workforce

Bliss, K. (2020). *Mental health and prison systems in major need of reform.* Prison Legal News. https://www.prisonlegalnews.org/news/2020/oct/1/mental-health-and-prison-systems-major-need-reform/

Boeree, G. (2006). *Carl Jung (1875–1961) personality theories.* Psychology Department Shippensburg University. https://webspace.ship.edu/cgboer/perscontents.html

Bradford, A. (2016). *Sigmund Freud: Life, work, & theories.* Live Science. http://www.live science.com

British Medical Journal. (2013). *People with mental illness at highly increased risk of being murder victims, study suggests.* Science Daily. https://www.sciencedaily.com/releases/2013/130305200455.htm

California Academy of Family Physicians. (2010). *CAFP launches family medicine initiative on trauma-informed care.* https://www.familydocs.org/aces

Canadian Agency for Drugs and Technologies in Health. (2014). *Delivery of electroconvulsive therapy in non-hospital settings: A review of the safety and guidelines.* https://www.ncbi.nlm.nih.gov/25520991

Canadian Centre on Substance Use and Addiction. (2021). *Mental health and substance use during COVID-19: Spotlight on youth, older adults & stigma.* https://www.ccsa.ca/mental-health-and-substance-use-during-covid-19

Carmona, J., Durand-Arias, S., Rodriguez, A., Guarner-Catala, C., Cardona-Muller, D., Madrigal-dé-Leon, E., & Alvarado, R. (2021). Community mental health care in Mexico: A regional perspective from a mid-income country. *International Journal of Mental Health Systems, 15*(7). https://doi.org/10.1186/s130330929099429-9

Cash, Mary, Cunnane, K., & Fan, C. (2020). Mapping cannabis potency in medical and recreational programs in the United States. *PLoSOne, 15*(3). e0230167. https://doi.org/10.137/journal.pone.0230167

Centers for Disease Control and Prevention. (2019). *Drug overdose deaths remain high.* U.S. Department of Health and Human services. https://www.cdc.gov/drugoverdose/deaths/index.html#

Centers for Disease Control and Prevention. (2022). *New CDC data illuminate youth mental health threats during COVID-19 pandemic.* U.S. Department of Health and Human Services. https://www.cdc.gov/media/releae/2022/p0331-youth-mental-health-covid-19.html

Centers for Disease Control and Prevention. (2021). Suicide prevention. https://www.cdc.gov/suicide/index.html

Centers for Medicare and Medicaid Services. (2021). *CMS data shows vulnerable Americans forgoing mental health care during COVID-19 pandemic.* https://www.cms.gov/newsroom/press-releases/cms-data-shows-vulnerable-americans-forgoing-mental-health-care-during-covid-19-pandemic

Center for Medicare and Medicaid Services. (2018). Inpatient psychiatric facility services Centers for Medicare and Medicaid Services. In *Medicare benefit policy manual* (Ch. 2, pp. 1–18).

Charpignon, M.L., Ontiveros, S., Sundaresan, S., Puri, A., Chandra, J., Mandl, K. D., & Majumder, M. S. (2022). Evaluation of suicides among adolescents during the COVID-19 pandemic. *JAMA Pediatr,* 176(7). 724–726. https://doi.org/10.1001/jamapediatrics.2022.0515. https://www/jamanetwork.com/journals/jamapediatrics/fullarticle/2791544

Columbia University Irving Medical Center. (2021). *How does COVID affect mental health?* https://www/cuimc.columbia.edu/news/how-does-covid-affect-mental-health

Corrigan, C., MBChB; Duke, G., MBBS, MD; Millar, J., MBChB, PhD; Paul, E., MSc, PhD; Butt, W., MBBS; Gordon, M., MBBS, MPM, MD; Coleman, J., MBBS; Pilcher, D., MBBS; Oberender, F., MBBS, PhD; for the Australian and New Zealand Intensive Care Society Pediatric Study Group (ANZICS PSG) and the ANZICS Center for Outcome and Resource Evaluation (ANZICS CORE). (2022). Admission of children and adolescents with deliberate self-harm to intensive care during the SARS-CoV-2 out-break in Australia. *JAMA Netw* (5), e 2211692. https://doi.org/10.1001/jamanetworkopen.2022.11692

Curwen, J., Nichols, C. H., Callender, J. H., & American Psychiatric Association. (1885). *Memoir of Thomas S. Kirkbride MD, LLD.* Direction of the Associates of Medical Superintendents of American Institution for the Insane. E. Rowan & Co.

D'Agostino, A., Demartini, B., Cavallotti, S., & Orsola, G. (2020). Mental Health Services in Italy during the COVID-19 outbreak. *The Lancet Psychiatry,* 7(5). https://doi.org/10.101016/S2215-0366(20)30133-4

de Bruin, T., & Robertson, G. (2019). Eugenics in Canada. In *The Canadian Encyclopedia.* https://www.thecanadianencyclopedia.ca.en/article/eugenics

Deutsche Welle Organization. (2018). U.S. and Colombia aim to halve cocaine production in five years. https://www.dw.com/en/us-and-colombia-aim-to-halve-cocaine-production-in-five-years/a-42793844

Devendorf, A., Rum, R., Kashdan, T. B., & Rottenberg, J. (2022). Optimal well-being after psychopathology: Prevalence and correlates. *Clinical Psychological Science.* https://doi.org/10.1177/21677026221078872

Deza, M., Maclean, J., & Solomon, K. (2020). *Local access to mental healthcare and crime.* https://www.nber.org/papers/w27619

Ding, J., & Hu, K. (2021). Cigarette smoking and schizophrenia: Etiology, clinical, pharmacological, treatment implications, *Hindawi* Schizophrenia Research and Treatment. 1–8. https://doi.org/10.1155/2021/769830

Drake, R., & Latimer, E. (2012). Lessons learned in developing community mental health in North America. *World Psychiatry, 11*(1), 47–51. https://doi.org/10.1016/j.wpsyc.2012.01.077

Drug-Free World. (2017). *How marijuana has changed over time.* https://www.drugfreeworld.org/course/lesson/the-truth-about-marijuana/its-background.html

Dziopa, F., & Ahern, K. (2008). What makes a quality therapeutic relationship in psychiatric/mental health nursing: A review of the research literature. *The Internet Journal of Advanced Nursing Practice, 10*(1). https://www.ispub.com/IJANP/10/1/7218

Eastern State Hospital. (n.d.). *America's first psychiatric hospital since 1773.* http://www.esh.dmhmrsas.virginia.gov/mission.html

eGyanKosh. (n.d.). *Historical development of psychiatric nursing.* https://www.egyankosh.ac.in/bitstream/123456789/31553/1/unit-1.pdf

Elflein, J. (2021). *Illicit drug use disorder among adults in the United States as of 2020, by level of mental illness.* https://www.statista.com/statistics/252473/us-iilicit-drug-dependence-or-abuse-by-level-of-mental-illness/

Esper, L. H., & Furtado, E. F. (2013). Gender differences and association between psychological stress and alcohol consumption: A systematic review. *J Alcoholism Drug Depend, 1*(116), 1–5. https://doi.org/10.4172/2329-6488.1000116

Faria, M. (2015). Neolithic trepanation decoded-A unifying hypothesis: Has the mystery as to why primitive surgeons performed cranial surgery been solved? *Surg Neurol Int, 6*, 72. https://doi.org/10.4103/2152-7806.156634

Faria, M. Jr. (2013). Violence, mental illness, and the brain-A brief history of psychosurgery: Part I-From trephination to lobotomy. *Surgical Neurology International,* 4, 49. https://doi.org/10.4103/2152-7806.110146, https://pubmed.ncbi.nlm.nih.gov/23646259

Fenollar-Cortés, J., Jiménez, Ó., Ruiz-García, A., & Resurrección, D.M. (2021). Gender differences in psychological impact of confinement during COVID-19 outbreak in Spain: A longitudinal study. *Front Psychol.* https://www.doi.org/10.3389/fpsyg.2021.682860

Fovet, T., Plancke, L., Amariei, A., Benradia, I., Carton, F., Sy, A., Kyheng, M., Tasniere, G., Amad, A., Danel, T., Thomas, P., & Roelandt, JL. (2020). Mental disorders on admission to jail: A study of prevalence and a comparison with community sample in the north of France. *Forensic Science International: Mind and Law.* https://journals.elsevier.com/forensic-science-international-mind-and-law

Franklin, M., & LaFee, S. (2021). *How adolescents used drugs during the COVID-19 pandemic.* UC San Diego Health. https://health.uscd/edu/news/releases/pages/2021-08-24/how-adolescents-used-drugs-during-the-covid-19-pandemic

Gaebel, W., & Zielasek, J. (2015). Homeless and mentally ill-a mental healthcare challenge for Europe. *Acta Psychiatr Scand.* 131(4), 236-8. https://doi.org/10.1111/acps.12394

Gaetz, S. (2012). *The real cost of homelessness: Can we save money by doing the right thing?* Homeless Hub Paper Series.

Gallant Law. (2019). *Mental illness and crime: What's the link?* https://www.gallantlaw.com.au/mental-illness-and-crime-whats-the-link/

Gazdag, G., Dragasek, J., Takács, R., Lõokene, M., Sobow, T., Olekseev, A., & Ungvari, G.S. (2017). Use of electroconvulsive therapy in Central-Eastern European countries: An overview. *Psychiatria Danubina, 29*(2), 136–140.

Ghaleb, Y., Lami, F., Al, Nsour M., Rashak, H.A., Samy, S., Khader, Y.S., Al Serouri, A., BahaaEldin. H., Afifi, S., Elfadul, M., Ikram, A., Akhtar, H., Hussein, A.M., Barkia, A., Hakim, H., Taha, H.A., Hijjo, Y., Kamal, E., Ahmed, A.Y., Rahman, F., Islam, K.M., Hussein, M.H., & Ramzi, S.R. (2021). Mental health impacts of COVID-19 on healthcare workers in the Eastern Mediterranean Region: A multi-country study. *Journal of Public Health, 43*(3), iii34–iii42. https://doi.org/10.1093/pubmed/fdab321

Giannis, D., Geropoulos, G., Matenoglou, E., & Moris, D. (2020). Impact of coronavirus disease 2019 on healthcare workers: Beyond the risk of exposure. *Postgraduate Medical Journal.* https://dx.doi.org/10.1136/postgradmedj-2020-137988

Gleckman, H. (2020). Why are so many nursing homes shutting down? *Forbes.* https://www.forbes.com/sites/howardgleckman/2020/03/02/why-are-so-many-nursing-homes-shutting-down/?sh=6d

Goslee, K. (2017). *Public health committee drills hospital administrator over alleged patient abuse.* FOX 61 news, https://www.fox61.com/article/news/local/outreach/awareness-months/public-hearing-monday-morning-on-alleged-abuse

Grabowski, D., Aschbrenner, KA., Rome, VF., & Bartels, SJ. (2010). Quality of mental health care for nursing home residents: A literature review. *Med Care Res Rev, 67*(6), 627–656. https://doi.org/10.1177/1077558710362538

Grigoletto, V., MD, Cognigni, M., MD, Agostino Occhipinti, A., MD, Abbracciavento, G., MD, Carrozzi, M., MD, Barbi, E., MD, PhD, & Cozzi, G., M.D. (2020). Rebound of severe alcoholic intoxications in adolescents and young adults after COVID-19 lockdown. *J Adolesc Health, 67*(5), 727–729. https://doi.org/10.1016/j.jadohealth.2020.08.017

Gutwinski, S. (2021). The prevalence of mental disorders among homeless people in high-income countries: An updated systematic review and meta-regression analysis. *PLoSMED, 23*(8), e1003750. https://doi.org/10.1371/journal.pmed.1003750, https://www.ncbi.nlm.nih.gov/pmc/articles/PMC8423293/

Harvard Health Publishing. (2014). *The homeless mentally ill.* Harvard Medical School. http://health.harvard.edu/newsletter_article/the_homeless_mentally_ill

Harvard Medical School. (2021). https://hms.harvard. edu/affiliates/mcclean-hospital

Hedegaard, H., Curtin, S.C., & Warner, M. (2018). *Suicide mortality in the United States, 1999–2017.* NCHS Data Brief, No. 330. National Center for Health Statistics, Center for Disease Control and Prevention. https://pubmed.ncbi.nlm.nih.gov/30500324/

Hung, P., Busch, S.H., Shih, Y.W., McGregor, A.J., & Wang, S. (2020). Changes in community mental health services availability and suicide mortality in the U.S.: A retrospective study. *BMC Psychiatry, 20,* 188, https://doi.org/10.1186/s12888-020-02607-y

Imtiaz, S., Nafeh, F., Russell, C., Ali, F., Elton-Marshall, T., & Rehm, J. (2021). The impact of the novel coronavirus disease (COVID-19) on drug overdose-related deaths in the United States and Canada: A systematic review of observational studies and analysis of public health surveillance data. *Substance Abuse Treatment, Prevention, and Policy, 16*(87). https://doi.org/10.1186/s13011-021-00423-5

International Association of Individual Psychology. (2012). *Alfred Adler.* https://www.adler.iaip.net

International Mental Health Collaborating Network. (2022). *24-7 community mental health centres.* https://www.imhcn.org/bibliography/recent-innovations-and-good-practices/community-mental-health-centres

Jeanroy, A. (n.d.). *Mental health laws in France.* European Community Based Mental Health Service Providers. https://www.eucoms.net/wp-content/uploads/2020/01/Laws-the-French-context-Aurora-Jeanroy-pdf

Jensen, P. (2015). Nursing. In *The Canadian Encyclopedia.* https://www.thecanadianencyclopedia.ca/en/article/nursing

Joint Commission on Administrative Rules, Administrative Code. Title 77, Public Health, Part 2060: Alcoholism and Substance Abuse Treatment and Intervention Licenses, Section 2060.401, levels of care, Section 2060.201.

Jones, S.E., Ethier, K.A., Hertz, M., DeGue, S., Le, V.D., Thornton, J., Lim, C., Dittus, P. J., Geda, S. (2022). Mental health, suicidality, and connectedness among high school students during the COVID-19 pandemic-adolescent behaviors and experiences survey, United States, January–June 2021. *United States Department of Health and Human Services, Center for Disease Control and Prevention, 71*(3), 16–21.

Kaelber, L., & Associate Professor of Sociology. (2012). *Eugenics: Compulsory sterilization in 50 American states.* University of Vermont. https://www.uvm.edu/-lkaelber/eugenics/

Kaelber, L. (2012). *Nebraska eugenics.* University of Vermont. http://www.uvm.edu/lkaelber/eugenics/NE/NE.html

Kaiser Family Foundation. (2022). *Adults reporting symptoms of anxiety or depressive disorder during COVID-19 pandemic.* https://www.kff.org/other/state-indicator/adults-reporting-symptoms-of-anxiety-or-depressive-disorder-during-covid-19-pandemic

Karki, A. (2018). Implementation of evidence-based care in mental health nursing: Barriers and strategies, https://www.thesus.fi/bitstream/handle/10024/166757/asmita%20-thesis.pdf?sequence=2

Keveney, B. (2021). More young children are killing themselves: The COVID-19 pandemic is making the problem worse. UC Irvine School of Medicine. *USA Today.* https://www.choc.org/news.more-young-children-are-killing-themselves-the-covid-19-pandemic-is-making-the-problem-worse

Kovner, J. (2017). 9 Arrested so far in patient abuse scandal at Whiting Forensic; 31 workers were suspended. *Hartford Courant.* https://www.courat.com/news/connecticut/hc-whiting-forensic-patient-abuse-arrests-0906-2017-0905-story.html

Kragh, J. (2010). Shock therapy in Danish psychiatry. Institute of Public Health. University of Copenhagen. *Medical History,* .(3), 341–364. https://doi.org/10.1017/s0025727300004646. https://europemc.org/aricle/MED/20592884

Kuntz, L., & Moutier, C. (2021). Breaking the trend: New CDC Data on suicide. *Psychiatric Times.* https://www.psychiatrictimes.com/view/breaking-the-trend-new-cdc-data-on-suicide

Laing Society. (2002). *R. D. Laing—biography.* http://www.laingsociety.org

Layman, H., Thorisdottir, I.E., Halldorsdottir, T., Sigfusdottir, I.D., Allegrante, J.P., & Kristjansson, A.L. (2022). Substance use among youth during the COVID-19 pandemic: A systematic review. *Curr Psychiatry Rep.* https://doi.org/10.1007/s11920-022-01338-z

Legal Action Center. (n.d.). *The Medicaid IMD exclusion: An overview and opportunities for reform.* http://lac.org/assets/files/IMD_exclusion_fact_sheet.pdf

Legal Information Institute. (n.d.). *Wyoming current rules and regulations for licensure of psychiatric hospitals.* https://www.law.cornell.edu/regulations/wyoming/agency

Leipzig University. (n.d.). *History of psychology in Leipzig, Germany.* Department of Psychology, http://www.psychologie.biphaps.uni-leipzig.de

Liu, S., Yang, L., Zhang, C., Xiang, Y.T., Liu, Z., Hu, S., & Zhang, B. (2020). Online mental health services in China during the COVID 19 outbreak. *The Lancet,* 7. https://doi.org/10.1016/S2215-0366(20)30077-8

Loewenstein, N. (2019). *The inappropriate institutionalization of people with mental illness in long-term care.* https://www.nuraunghome411.org/wp-content/uploads/2021/02/webinar.institutionalization.02162021.pdf

Luciano, A., & Meara, E. (2014). The employment status of people with mental illness: National survey data from 2009–2010. *Psychiatric Serv, 65*(10), 1201–1209. https://doi.org/10.1176/appi. ps.201300335

Lyon, E. (2019). *Imprisoning America's mentally ill.* Prison Legal News. https://www.prisonlegalnews.org2019/feb/4/imprisoning-americas-mentally-ill

MacQueen, G. (2007). The long-term impact of treatment with electroconvulsive therapy on discrete memory systems in patients with bipolar disorder. *Journal of Psychiatry and Neuroscience, 32*(4), 241–249

Makeenko, V. (2020). *Mombello Psychiatric Hospital.* Abandoned Spaces. https://www.abandonedspaces.com/hospital/mombello-psychiatric-hospital.html?edg-c=1

Marcus, L., Johnson, C., & Ramirez, D. (2021). The complex link between homelessness and mental illness. *Psychology Today.* https://psychologytoday.com/us/blog/mind-matters-menninger/202105/the-complex-link-between-homelessness-and-mental-illness

McBratney, L. (2022). Victimization of people with mental illness. *Trauma and Victimization—Visions Journal, 3*(3), 8–9. https://www.heretohelp.bc.ca/victimization-people-mental-illness

Mental Health America. (2021). *Mental health and COVID-19.* https://mhanational.org/mental-health-and-covid-19

Mental Health Foundation. (2022). *eMEN digital mental health European project.* https://cpmr.mentalhealth.org.uk/sp/node/2092

Mental Health Services for Children and Adolescents (n.d.). *Family guide: Children's mental health services.* Texas Department of State Health Services. http://www.dshs.state.tx.us/mhsa/mh-child-adolescent-services.

Mental Illness Policy. (2012). *New study suggests that severely mentally ill individuals who are not being treated are responsible for 10 percent of U.S. homicides.* https://www.mentalillnesspolicy.org/consequences/1000-homicides.html

Morant, N., Kaminskiy, E., & Ramon, S. (2016). Shared decision making for psychiatric medication management: Beyond the micro-social. *Health Expectations: An International Journal of Public Participation in Health Care and Health Policy, 19*(5), 1002–1014. https://doi.org/10.111/hex.12392

Moroz, N., Moroz, I., & D'Angelo, M.S. (2020). Mental health services in Canada: Barriers and cost-effective solutions to increase access. *Healthc Manage Forum.* 33(6), 282–287. https://doi.org/10.1177/0840470420933911

National Alliance on Mental Illness. (2022). *Crisis intervention team (CIT) programs.* https://www.nami.org/advocacy/crisis-intervention/crisis-intervention-team-programs

National Alliance on Mental Illness. (2022). Crisis response. https://www.nami.org/advocacy/policy-priorities/responding-to-crisis/crisis-response

National Alliance on Mental Illness. (2021). *Mental health treatment while incarcerated.* https://www.nami.org/advocacy/policy-priorities/improving-health/mental-health-treatment-while-incarcerated

National Alliance on Mental Illness. (2021). *What you need to know about the cost and accessibility of mental health care in America.* https://www.nami.org/press-media/in-the-news/2021/what-you-need-to-know-about-the-cost-and-accessibility-of-mental-health-care-in-america

National Center for Health Statistics. (2022). *U.S. overdose deaths in 2021 increased half as much in 2020—but are still up 15%.* Center for Disease Control and Prevention. https://www.cdc.gov/nchs/pressroom/nchs_press_releases/2022/202205.htm

National Commission on Correctional Healthcare. (2021). *Basic mental health services.* https://www.ncchc.org/spotlight-on-the-standards/basic-mental-health-services

National Council on Behavioral Health. (2020). *How to manage trauma.* https://www. thenationalcouncil.org/resources/how-to-manage-trauma/

National Institute of Health. (2021). *Why is there comorbidity between substance use disorders and mental illness?* https://www.drugabuse.gov/publications/research-reports/common-comorbities-substance-use

National Institute on Drug Abuse. (2010). Comorbidity: Addiction and other mental illness. *Research Reports.* https://drugabuse.gov/publications/research-reports/comorbidity-addiction-other-mental-illness

National Institute on Drug Abuse. (2021). *Marijuana: Is there a link between marijuana use and psychiatric disorders?* https://www.drugabuse.gov/publications/research-reports/marijuana

National Institute on Drug Abuse. (2021). *What are the treatments for comorbid substance use disorder and mental health conditions?* https://www.drugabuse.gov

Nochaiwong, S., Ruengorn, C., Thavorn, K., Hutton, B., Awiphan, R., Phosuya, C., Ruanta, Y., Wongpakaran, N., Wongpakaran, T. (2021). Global prevalence of mental health issues among the general population during the coronavirus disease-2019 pandemic: a systematic review and meta-analysis. *Sci Rep, 11,* 10173, https://doi.org/10.1038/s41598-021-89700-8

Nuland, S. (2011). Sigmund Freud's cocaine years. *New York Times.* https://www.nytimes.com/2011/07/24/book/review/an-anatomy-of-addiction-by-howard-markel/html

Nursing Home Abuse Justice. (2022). *Mental health in nursing homes: Managing emotional health.* https://www.nursinghomeabuse.org/resources/nursing-home-mental-health

Olsen, D. (2022). *We explain how to access different mental health services in Germany, as well as private health insurance, emergency support, and more.* https://www.expatica.com/de/healthcare-services/mental-health-in-germany-346138

Opacity. (n.d). Pilgrim State Hospital, Abandoned Photography. http://opacity.us/site23_pilgrim_state_hospital.htm.

Open Minds. (2019). *The connection between homelessness and mental health.* https://www.openminds.org.au/news/the-connection-between-homelessness-and-mental-health

Orth, J., Li, Y, Simning, A., Temkin-Greener, H. (2019). Providing behavioral health services in nursing homes is difficult: Findings from a national survey. *Journal of American Geriatrics Society, 67*(8), 1713–1717. https://pubmed.ncbi.nlm.nih.gov/31166614

Panchal, N., Kamal, R., Cox, C., Garfield, R., & Chidambaram, P. (2021). *Mental health and substance use considerations among children during the COVID-19 pandemic.* Kaiser Family Foundation. https://www.kff.org/blog/mental-health-and-substance-use-among-children-during-the-covid-19-pandemic

Panchal, N., Saunders, H., Rudowitz, R., & Cox, C. (2021). *The implications of COVID-19 for mental health and substance use.* Kaiser Family Foundation, https://www.kff.org/coronavirus-covid-19/issue-brief/the-implications-of-covid-19-for-mental-health-and-substance-use/

Patterson, E. (n.d.). *Dual diagnosis substance abuse and mental illness treatment. Mental health and drug abuse.* http://www.drugabuse.com/mental-health-drug-abuse

Paul, E., & Fancourt, D. (2022). Factors influencing self-harm thoughts and behaviors over the first year of the COVID-19 pandemic in the UK: Longitudinal analysis of 49,324 adults. *Br J Psychiatry*, (1), 31–37. https://doi.org/10.1192/bip.2021.130

Pedersen, B., & Kolstad, A. (2009). De-institutionalization and trans-institutionalization-changing trends of inpatient care in Norwegian mental health institutions 1950–2007. *International Journal of Mental Health Systems, 3*, 28. https://doi.org/10.1186/1752-4458-3-28, https://pubmed.ncbi.nlm.nih.gov/200356231/

Peltier, M., Verplaetse, T.L., Mineur, Y.S., Petrakis, I.L., Cosgrove, K.P., Picciotto, M.R., & McKee, S.A. (2019). Sex differences in stress-related alcohol use. *Neurobiol Stress, 10*, 100149. https://doi.org/10.1016/j.ynstr.2019.100149. https://pubmed,ncbi.nlm.nih. gov/309495621/

Phillips, A. (1978). *The role of nursing homes in the deinstitutionalization of psychiatric patients from state hospitals.* https://www.scholarworks.umass.edudissertation_1/3431/#

Placzek, J. (2016). *Did the emptying of mental hospitals contribute to the homelessness?* https://www.kqed.org/news/11209729/did-the-emptying-of-mental-hospitaks-contribute-to-homelessness

Prins, S., (2014). *Prevalence of mental illness in U.S. state prisons: A systematic review.* https://doi.org/10.1176/appi.ps.201.30066

Racine, N., McArthur, B.A., Cooke, J.E., Eirich, R., Zhu, J., Madigan, S. (2021). Global prevalence of depressive and anxiety symptoms in children and adolescents during COVID-19. *JAMA Pediatric, 175*(11), 1142–1150. https://doi.org/10.1001/jama-pediatrics.2021.2482

Raphael, S., & Stoll, M. (2014). Assessing the contribution of the deinstitutionalization of the mentally ill to growth in the U.S. Incarceration Rate. *The Journal of Legal Studies, 42*(1), 187–222.

Recovery Connection. (2011). *Addiction treatment modalities and programs.* https://www.recoveryconnection.com

Reilly, P. (2015). Eugenics and involuntary sterilization: 1907–2015. *Annu Rev Genomics Hum Genet. 16*, 351–368. https://doi.org/10.1146/annurev-genom-090314-024930

Resnick, B. (2021). *Psychiatrists are uncovering connections between viruses and mental health.* Voxmedia. https://www.vox.com/science-and-health/227883685/covid-19-depression-mental-health-risks-immunology

Robeznieks, A. (2015). *Mental health workforce shortage a worldwide issue.* Modern Healthcare. https://wwwmodernhealthcare.com/article/20150715/news/150719943/mental-health-workforce-shortage-a-worldwide-issue#

Robeznieks, A. (2021). *Why doctors must grasp patient's context in trauma-informed care.* AMA. https://www.ama-assn.org/delivering-care/health-equity/why-doctors-must-grasp-patients-contex-in-trauma-informed-care

Rogers, C. (2014). *Inside the world's most dangerous hospital.* BBC News. https://www.bbc.com/news/magazine-30293880

Roots Community Health Center. (2021). How much would it cost to end homelessness in America? https://rootsclinic.org/how-much-would-it-cost-to-end-homelessness-in-america

Rossiter, K., & Clarkson, A. (2013). Opening Ontario's saddest chapter: A social history of Huronia Regional Centre. *Canadian Journal of Disability Studies, 2*(3), 1–30. https://doi.org/10.15353/cjds.v2i3.99.

S.1177-Mental Health Systems Act. 96th Congress (1979–1980). https://www.congress.gov/bill/96th-congress/senate-bill/1177

Sainty, L. (2018). *Two doctors connected to the deep sleep therapy medical scandal are suing over an ABC journalist's scientology book.* Buzzfeed. https://www.buzzfeed.com/lanesainty/two-doctors-connected-to-the-deep-sleep-therapy-medical

Scaly, P., & Whitehead, P. (2004). Forty years of deinstitutionalization of psychiatric services in Canada: An Empirical Assessment. *Can J Psychiatry, 49*(4), 250.

Schanda, H., Stompe, T., & Ortwein-Swoboda, G. (2009). Dangerous or merely difficult? The new population of forensic mental hospitals. *European Psychiatry, 24*(6), 365–372. https://doi.org/10.1016/j.eurpsy.2009.07.006

Schillo, K. (2011). *Nature or nurture: The case of the boy who became a girl.* National Center for Case Study Teaching in Science. https://sciencecases.lib.buffalo.edu/files/gender-reassignent.pdf

Schluter, P., Généreux, M., Hung, K.K., Landaverde, E., Law, R.P., Mok, C.P.Y., Murray, V., O'Sullivan, T., Qadar, Z., & Roy, M. (2022). Patterns of suicidal ideation across eight countries in four continents during the COVID-19 pandemic era: Repeated cross-sectional study. *JMIR Public Health Surveill, 8*(1), e32140. https://doi.org/10.2196/32140

Scholl L., Seth, P., Kariisa, M., Wilson, N., & Baldwin, G. (2018). Drug and opioid-involved overdose deaths United States, 2013–2017. *Morbidity and Mortality Weekly Report, 67*(5152), 1419–1427. https://dx.doi.org/10.15585/mmwr.mm6751e

Schreiter, S., Bermpohl, F., Krausz, M., Leucht, S., Rössler, W., Schouler-Ocak, M., & Gutwinski, S. (2017). The prevalence of mental illness in homeless people in Germany. *Dtsch Arztebl Int, 114*(40), 665–672. https://doi.org/10.3238/arztebl.2017.0665

Schwarzwalder, A. (2017). Mental disorder and crime. Crime and Law. https://wwwantonio-casella.eu

Seattle School of Law. (2018). *The effectiveness of housing first and permanent supportive housing.* https://www.law.seattle.edu/doc/5941324/the-effectiveness-of-housing-first-and-permanent-supportive-housing

Shaw, L., & Kurbegovic, E. (2014). *Sweden.* Eugenic Archives. https://www. eugenicsarchive.ca/discover/tree/51c27497b894oa54000009

Sherman, L., Lynch, S.E., Teich, J., & Hudock, W.J. (2017). Availability of supported employment in specialty mental health treatment facilities and facility characteristics: 2014. *The CBHSQ Report.* Substance Abuse and Mental Health Services Administration.

Sinclair, E. (2018). Research weekly: *Violence in hospitals by people with serious mental illness.* Treatment Advocacy Center. https://advocacycenter.org/fixing-the-system/features-and-news

Society for Recognition of Famous People. (2020). *The famous people: Psychiatrists.* http://the-famouspeople.com/psychiatrists.php

Society of Personality Assessment. (2005). The status of the Rorschach in clinical and forensic practice: An official statement by the Board of Trustees of the Society for personality testing. *Journal of Personality Assessment, 85*(2), 219–237.

Sorbo, E. (2016). Ruins of memory: A sustainable conservation for the material and immaterial values of the former psychiatric hospitals in Italy. *Procedia Engineering.* 161, 2198–2202 https://doi:10.1016/proeng.2016.08.815

Spanko, A. (2019). *Even as demands rises, nursing homes face major behavioral health hurdles.* Skilled Nursing News. https://www.skillednursingnews.com.2019/06/depite-demands-nursing-homes-face-major-behavioral-health-hurdles

Srivastava, P., & Panday, R. (2017). Psychoeducation an effective tool as treatment 2 modality in mental health. *The International Journal of Indian Psychology, 4*(1), 123–130. DIP: 18.01.153/20160401.

State of California. (2021). California Department of State Hospitals–Napa. https://www.dsh.ca.gov/napa

Stegge, G.J. (2004). Psychiatric training of nurses in the Netherlands since 1883. *Gewina, 27*(2), 78–99. https://www.pubmed.ncbi.nim.nih.gov/15359463/

Substance Abuse and Mental Health Services Administration. (2021). *Key substance use and mental health indicators in the United States: Results from the 2020 national survey on drug use and health* (HHS Publication No. PEP21-07-01-003, NSDUH Series H-56). Center for Behavioral Health Statistics and Quality, http://www.samhsa.gov/data/sites/default/reports/rpt353191/2020NSDUHFFR1PDFW102121.pdf

Substance Abuse and Mental Health Services Administration. (2009). *Illness and management recovery*, No. SMA-09-4462. U.S. Department of Health and Human Services.

Substance Abuse and Mental Health Services Administration. (2009). *Integrated treatment for co-occurring disorders*, No. SMA-08-4366. U.S. Department of Health and Human Services.

Substance Abuse and Mental Health Services Administration. (2014). https://samhsa.gov

Sweeney, C., Potts, C., Ennis, E., Bond, R., Mulvenna, M., O'Neill, S., Malcolm, M., Kuosmanen, L., Kostenius, C., Vakaloudis, A., McConvey, G., Urkington, R., Hanna, D., Nieminen, H., Vartianen, A.K., Robertson, A., & McTear, M. (2021). Can chatbots help support a person's mental health? Perceptions and views from mental healthcare professionals and experts. *ACM Trans. Comp. Healthcare, 2*(3). https://doi.org/10.1145/3453175

Sylvestre, M.P., Dinkou, G.D.T., Naja, M., Riglea, T., Pelekanakis, A., Bélanger, M., Maximova, K., Mowat, D., Paradis, G., & O'Loughlin, J. (2022). A longitudinal study of change in substance use from before to during the COVID-19 pandemic in young adults. *The Lancet Regional Health, 8*, 100168. https://doi.org/10.1016/j.lana.2021.100168

Tabler, D. (2008). *125 reasons you'll get sent to the lunatic asylum*. Appalachian History. https://apalachianhistory.net/2008/12/125-reasons-youll-get-sent-to-lunatic-html

Teplin, L., McClelland, G.M., Abram, K.M., & Weiner, D.A. (2006). Crime victimization in adults with severe mental illness. *Arch Gen Psychiatry, 62*(8), 911–921. https://doi.org/10.1001/archpsyc.62.8.911

The Daily Dose, (n.d.). May 5, 1817: Founding of the Friends Asylum for the Relief of Persons Deprived of the Use of Their Reason. https://www.awb.com/dailydose/?p=1196

The Extra Mile-Points of Light Volunteer Pathway, (n.d). Clifford W. Beers. https://www.extra-mile.us/honorees/beers.cfm

The Lewin Group. (2004). *Costs of serving homeless individuals in nine cities*. Chart Book.

Thornicroft, G., Deb, T., & Henderson, C. (2016). Community mental health care worldwide: current status and further developments. *World Psychiatry, 15*(3), 276–286. https://doi.org/10.1002/wps.20349

The White House. (2023). *Fact sheet: Biden-Harris administration announces new actions to tackle nation's mental health crisis*. https://www.whitehouse.gov/briefing-room/statements-releases/2023/05/18/fact-sheet-biden-harris-administration-announces-new-actions-to-tackle-nations-mental-health-crisis/

Thornicroft, G., & Tansella, M. (2013). The balanced care model: The case for both hospital-and community-based mental healthcare. *Br J Psychiatry, 102*(4), 246–248. https://doi.org/10.1192/bjp.bp.112.111377

Sen, L.T., Siste, K., Hanafi, E., Murtani, B.J., Christian, H., Limawan, A.P., & Adrian, Siswidiani, L.P. (2021). Insights into adolescents' substance use in a low-middle-income country during the COVID-19 pandemic. *Front Psychiatry, 14*, https://doi.org/10.3389/fpsyt.2021.739698

Tiao, J. (n.d.). *The history of Bethlem Hospital*. Hektoen International. https://www.hekint.org/2017/02/22/the-history-of-bethlem-hospital/

Tikkanen, R., Osborn, R., Mossialos, E., Djordjevic, A., & Wharton, G. (2020). *International health care system profiles, Italy*. Commonwealth Fund. https://www. commonwealthfund.org/international-health-policy-center/countries/Italy

Treatment Advocacy Center. (2019). *Research weekly: Beyond road runners: Insights from other countries.* https://wwwtreatmentadvocacycenter.org/fixing-the-system/features-and-news/4168-research-weekly-beyond-road-runners

UNICEF. (2021). *Community-based mental health care in Peru.* https://www.unicef.org/stories/community-based-mental-health-care-in-peru

UNICEF. (2021). *On my mind: Promoting, protecting, and caring for children's mental health. The state of the world's children.* https://www.unicef.org/yemen/media/5806/file/the-state-of-the-worlds-children-report.pdf

UNICEF. (2020). *The impact of COVID-19 on the mental health of adolescents and youth.* https://www.unicef.org/lac/en/impact-covid-19-mental-health-adolescents-and-youth

United Nations Office on Drugs and Crime. (2021). COVID-19 and drugs: Impact outlook, No. E.21.XL.8. *World Drug Report 2021.*

University of North Dakota. (2022). *What is community mental health.* https://www.onlinedegrees.und.edu

U.S. Legal (n.d.). *Supported employment laws and legal definition.* https://definitions.uslegal.com/s/supported-employment/

Unutzer, J., MD, MPH, Harbin, H., MD, Schoenbaum, M., PhD, & Druss, B., MD, MPH. (2013). The collaborative care model: An approach for integrating physical and mental health care in Medicaid health homes. https://www.chcs.org/resource/the-collaborative-care-model-an-approach-for-integrating-physical-and-mental-health-care-in-medicaid-health-homes

van der Schaaf, P.S., Dusseldorp, E., Keuning, F.M., Janssen, W.A., & Noorthoorn, E.O. (2013). Impact of the physical environment of psychiatric wards on the use of seclusion. *The British Journal of Psychiatry,* 1–6.

Velligan, D., Sajatovic, M., Hatch, A., Kramata, P., & Docherty, J.P. (2017). Why do psychiatric patients stop antipsychotic medications? A systemic review of reasons for non-adherence to medication in patients with serious mental illness. *Dove Press, 11,* 449–468. https://doi.org/10.2147/PPA.S124658

Wagner, S. (2012). *State hospitals are still snake pits of patient abuse, betrayal of the public.* Psychiatric Crime Database. https://www.psychcrime.org/articles/index.php?vd=12

Walsh, S. (2018). *FDA in brief: FDA takes action to ensure regulation of electroconvulsive therapy devices better protects patients, reflects current understanding of safety and effectiveness.* U.S Department of Health and Human Services, Food and Drug Administration, Center for Devices and Radiological. https://www.fda.gov/news-events/fda-brief/fda-brief-fda-takes-action-to-ensure-regulation-of-electroconvulsive-therapy-devices

Weltens, I., Bak, M., Verhagen, S., Vandenberk, E., Domen, P., van Amelsvoort, T., & Drukker, M. (2021). Aggression on the psychiatric ward: Prevalence and risk factors. A systematic review of the literature. *PLoS One, 18*(10), e0258346. https://doi.org/10.1371/journal.pone.0268346. https://pubmed.ncbi.nlm.nih.gov/34624057

Wiegand, H., Bröcker, A.L., Fehr, M., Lohmann, N., Maicher, B., Röthke, N., Rueb, M., Wessels, P., de Greck, M., Pfennig, A., Unterecker, S., Tüscher, O., Walter, H., Falkai, P., Lieb, K., Hölzel, L.P., & Adorjan, K. (2022). Changes and challenges in inpatient mental health care during the first two high incidence phases of the COVID-19 pandemic in Germany—results from COVID psychiatry survey. *Front Psychiatry.* https://doi.org/10.3389/fpsyt.2022.855040

Wikipedia. (n.d.). *Psychiatric and mental health nursing.* http://en.wikipedia.org/wiki/psychiatric_and_mental_health_nursing

Wilkinson, S., Agbese, E., Leslie, D.L., & Rosenheck, R.A. (2018). Identifying recipients of electroconvulsive therapy: Data from privately insured Americans. *Psyciatr Serv, 69*(5), 542–548. https://doi.org/10.1176/appi.ps.201700364. https://www.ncbi.nlm.nih.gov/29385954

Williams, B. (2020). *Q & A with former APA President Dr. Steven Sharfstein: Suicides and psychiatric beds.* https://psychiatryadvisor.com/home/topics/suicide-and-self-harm/qa-with-former-apa-president-dr-steven-sharfstein

Wong Hoi-Ching, B., Chkonia, E., Pinchuk, I., Panteleeva, L., Stevanovic, Tufan, A.E., Skokauskas, N., & Ougrin, D. (2022). Transitioning to community-based mental healthcare: Reform experiences of five countries. *BiPsych International, 19*(1), 18–21.

World Health Organization. (2020). *COVID-19 disrupting mental health services in most countries, WHO survey.* https://www.who.int/news/item/5-10-2020/c ovid-19-disrupting-mental-health-services-in-most-countries-who-survey

World Health Organization. (2014). *Mental health: A state of well-being.* https://www.who.int/factfiles/mental_health/en

World Health Organization. (2022). Mental health and COVID-19: Early evidence of the pandemic's impact. *Scientific Brief.* https://www.apps.who.int/publications/i/item/who-2019-ncov-sci_briefmental_health-2022.1

World Health Organization. (2021). *Mental health: WHO special initiative for mental health.* https://www.who.int/intiatives/who-special-initiative-for-mental-health

World Health Organization. (2021). *New WHO guidance seeks to put an end to human rights violations in mental health care.* https://www.who.int/news/item/10-06-2021-new-whos-guidance-seeks-to-put-an-end-to-human-rights-violations-in-mental-health-care

World Population Review. (2022). Countries with universal health care 2022. https://www.worldpopulationreview.com/country-ranking/countries-with-universal-health-care

Xiao, J., Wang, R., Hu, Y., He, T., Ruan, Z., Chen, Q., & Peng, Z. (2022). Impacts of psychological stress response on non-suicidal self-injury during the COVID-19 epidemic in China: The medication role of sleep disorders. *BMC Psychology, 10*(87). https://doi.org/10.1186/s40359-022-00789-6

Zerrin, A. (2012). Cannabis, a complex plant: Different compounds and different effects on individuals. *Ther Adv Psychopharmacol, 2*(6), 241–254. https://doi.org/10.1177/2045125312457586

Zhoa, S., Sampson, S,. Xia, J., & Jayaram, M.B. (2015). Psychoeducation (brief) for people with serious mental illness. *Cochrane Database of Systematic Reviews, 4,* 1. https://doi.org/10.1002/14651858

Zhong, B.L., Zhou, D.Y., He, M.F., Li, Y., Li, W.T., Ng, C.H., Xiang, Y.T., & Chiu, H.F. (2020). Mental health problems, needs, and service use among peope living within and outside Wuhan during the COVID-19 epidemic in China. *Annals of Translational Medicine, 8*(21), 1392. https://doi.org/10.21057/atm02904145

Zimmer, Z., Rojo, F., Ofstedal, M.B., Chiu, C.T., Saito, Y., & Jagger, C. (2019). Religiosity and health: A global comparative study. *SSM Popul Health,* 100322, 7. https://doi.org/10.1016/j.ssmph.2018.11.006

INDEX

N

O

P

Q

R

S

T

U

W

www.ingramcontent.com/pod-product-compliance
Ingram Content Group UK Ltd.
Pitfield, Milton Keynes, MK11 3LW, UK
UKHW050141280726
14058UKWH00006B/759

9 798823 329712